The Lymph

Dr. Angela Fetzner

Translated by Phil Stanway

"The Lymph"
Written By Dr. Angela Fetzner

Distributed by Babelcube, Inc.
www.babelcube.com
Translated by Phil Stanway
Cover Design © 2020 ZERO agency munich germany using motives from shutterstock.com - Picture © IvaFoto shutterstock.com

Contents

Lymphatic cleansing

This has become the stepchild of all detoxification therapy. Cleansing of the liver or colon is high on the agenda, but detoxification of the lymphatic system is often neglected. Regular detoxification of the lymphatic system is nonetheless crucial for physical and mental health.

The lymphatic system

This is the body's purification plant, ridding it of whatever is harmful or useless like pathogens, metabolic waste, toxins and cell debris. It is crucial for immunity and the body's detoxification.

Sustaining the flow

The lymphatic system must be regularly cleansed and detoxified to keep on flowing naturally. If continually overloaded with waste, it stagnates. The system can no longer get rid of all problematic materials, so these gradually poison the whole body and often cause chronic ailments.

Lymphatic cleansing

This book outlines all natural therapies and treatments which have proven to be effective in basic lymphatic detoxification and cleansing. These everyday ways to look after yourself are motivating and efficient. They include approaches like medicinal plant therapy, homeopathy, Schuessler salts, specific cleansing of the lymph, water applications, stress reduction, changes of diet, moderate exercise and so on. With the help of these choice means of detoxification, you will soon feel livelier, stronger and merrier.

As a doctor of pharmacology, the author has been advising and informing clients for more than two decades, being committed to their health and well being.

Your pharmacist, Angela Fetzner

Cleansing by the lymphatic system

While cleansing of the liver or colon is high on the agenda of any detoxification therapy, the same is not true of detoxification of the lymphatic system. This is surely due to he fact that this system works mainly out of sight so is one of the more neglected parts of the body. Mostly, we pay attention to it only when the child has already fallen into the well, but many ailments are not even properly diagnosed as being due to an impaired flow of lymph.

Moreover, all measures for cleansing the gut or liver remain ineffective or even counterproductive if the lymphatic system is already overloaded. They only overload the system further, which is one of the most common and ominous mistakes made in the course of detoxification. The role of the lymphatic system in detoxification is thus very important, as it is responsible for destroying and removing pollutants (chemicals, traces of medicines, toxins, wastes, old and unusable cells, cell debris, cancerous cells, bacteria and viruses) isolated by our immune cells. Any kind of detoxification should always include stimulation of the lymphatic system, as stimulating the flow of lymph facilitates the removal of metabolic end products, toxins and pathogens.

The lymph system can rightly be called the body's purification system because, if the filtration no longer works well, the body becomes polluted with toxins, bacteria, viruses, fungi, cell debris, slag and dysfunctional cells. Needless to say, this augers the beginning of many ailments acute and chronic. Moreover, due to lymphatic drainage, cells can no longer be supplied with enough nutrients. Hence holistic lymphatic cleansing is one of the most important measures for preventing or healing ailments of all kinds, for only through continuous purification is the body's water kept wonderfully clean and healthy.

The lymphatic system should also be credited with taking on even coarse and unwieldy waste. Its capillaries absorb bacteria, bacterial toxins, viruses, fungi, heavy metals, chemicals, cell debris, dysfunctional and degenerate cells and bear them as highly toxic waste in the lymph fluid to the lymph nodes, where the concentrated waste is finally filtered and detoxified. The lymph nodes render all kinds of pollutants harmless then send the purified lymph into the blood stream. It should no longer be surprising that our health depends so crucially on the performance of the lymphatic system, as it acts as the police force and guardian of our health.

The lymph nodes are packed with phagocytes and lymphocytes, which eagerly destroy bacteria and literally feast on cancer cells. Given this range of responsibilities, the system is continuously dealing with waste of all kinds like toxins, bacteria, viruses, parasites, fungi, slags, mucilage and degenerate cells. Even waste too toxic for other organs to deal with is patiently accepted by the lymphatic system.

However, if this system is continually overworked and the lymphatic activity is inadequately stimulated, the efficiency of the lymph nodes or of the immune cells and phagocytes within them declines. The lymph becomes sluggish and begins to accumulate. The result can be suitably likened to a stagnant body of water with poison seeping into it. The river is blocked, the poison accumulates and the river dies. This image is drastic but hardly exaggerated. If the lymphatic system is overloaded, toxins and slag from the lymphatic fluid can enter the bloodstream, and the body be slowly but surely poisoned.

Such a blockage may cause numerous complaints like swollen eyes, thick legs and also cellulite. There may be an odd but leaden fatigue, a decline in our efficiency, a weakness in concentrating, a chronic headache, sundry aches and pains, recurrent colds, chronic sinus infections, allergies, acne and menstrual cramps. In the long run, there may even be severe chronic ailments like cancer.

The lymph system is not only responsible for detoxification but, along with the gut, is also the most important part of our immune system, so a holistic purification of the lymph can hardly receive too much attention.

The lymphatic system also has a special feature, which makes a regular detoxification even more important. Its vessels run next to and alongside those of the circulatory system for the blood. But significantly, whereas the circulatory system is driven by the heart's pump, there is no pump driving fluid though the lymphatic system. Instead, the system relies on external activation, to which we should now pay attention.

An adequate flow of lymph is also very important because of the slow rate of flow. Only 1.5 to 2.5 l of lymph flow through the lymphatic vessels per day, whereas about 5.0 l of blood (the body's total amount) flow through the blood vessels per minute.

Cleansing of the lymphatic system

Since the lymph does not flow of its own accord, it must be stimulated and activated, to let it be fast and unimpaired, then slag, pathogens, cancer cells and toxins can quickly and effectively pass out of the body. Stimulating the lymphatic activity also avoids the dreaded lymphatic blockage.

Likewise the other detoxifying organs should be relieved and cleansed, to let the lymphatic system devote itself now and then to regeneration. Ultimately the lymphatic system benefits from a cleansing and detoxification of the liver, intestine and kidneys, because if the other detoxifying organs are contaminated with pollutants, it too is likely to suffer. The other detoxifying organs are only too happy to pass waste on to the lymphatic system.

But before we can get a clear idea of how to keep it healthy, we should look more generally at all aspects of detoxification of the body.

The boons of detoxification

Detoxification – the removal of pollutants from the body – has a long past. Since time immemorial, people have wished to cleanse themselves, body and soul, on a regular basis, to remove all needless and harmful ballast. This wish may have been due to an instinctive feeling that purification is a great relief for body and soul and is also needed to maintain or regain health. A thorough detoxification and cleansing of the body is also a precondition for all deeper processes of healing.

Detoxification measures may also serve to activate the self-healing powers of the body, because only if the body is thoroughly freed from pollutants are many ailments deprived of a substrate, letting body and soul recover. The pollutants may consist of the body's own metabolic residues and acids, mold, organic solvents, heavy metals, formaldehyde, dioxin, radioactivity and so on. Of course, not only the body but also the mind has pollutants in the form of traumatic experiences, fears or unprocessed problems.

Such pollutants needlessly hinder and weaken us and finally make us ill, so body and soul should be freed from the load. Otherwise countless environmental toxins and other pollutants lessen our physical and mental resilience and cause us to ail in many ways. Here careful detoxification and cleansing treatment can usefully be applied, especially if several detoxification measures are combined, to let more be achieved. Diverse measures may deeply and finely aid and abet one another but only if they are precisely coordinated. The processes of cleansing may then serve to activate self-healing powers and to harmonize misdirected energies within the body.

Not surprisingly, after such treatment we may feel reborn and free. If mind, body and soul have been thoroughly cleansed and regenerated through detoxification, we may feel deeply relaxed, brimming with joy and vitality and be able to cope more efficiently with everyday life. If the detoxification cure is given ample time, space and attention, the positive changes may be deep and lasting.

Many complaints such as continual weariness, fatigue, insomnia and lack of energy completely disappear or lastingly improve. Also the gastrointestinal tract benefits from thorough cleansing of the body, so complaints such as constipation, fullness, bloating, heartburn and nausea are soon relegated to the past. A careful cleansing of the body also improves allergies and skin diseases such as impure skin, eczema and poorly healing wounds. Detoxification also improves pains in the joints or elsewhere and every kind of inflammation.

The mind too benefits from thorough detoxification, as nervousness and inner restlessness often vanish, and depression and anxiety are often greatly alleviated. A cleansing of the body also freshens the mind, especially the powers of concentration and memory, and last but not least, a detoxification of the body often impressively reduces obesity.

Renewing cells in general through detoxification also benefits skin and hair, letting a person look years younger, but the benefit extends to other organs. This is especially true of such organs of detoxification as the liver, kidneys, skin and lungs as well as the lymphatic system, as they all become more active and efficient.

Thorough detoxification is also the basic prerequisite for vitality, well-being and dynamism as well as being the first and foremost step towards the healing of ailments of all kinds. Indeed, naturopathy ascribes all ailments to pollutants affecting the body and mind. Sustainable detoxification activates the body's self-healing powers, prompting it to follow the path of healing of its own accord to the goal of complete recovery.

But a stitch in time saves nine, so detoxification is also recommended for people apparently healthy, whose vitality and quality of life may be further increased. Such cleansing hinders the process of aging, increasing both mental and physical reliance, and tones the immune system up, lessening the frequency of colds and infections. This route to a healthier way of life can also be smoothed by limiting or abandoning smoking and alcohol.

Health & detoxification

Thorough detoxification is the basis of health and also the precondition for curing ailments of all kinds. If the body is not regularly detoxified, the overload of toxins and slags gradually becomes too great to be adequately disposed of and these troublemakers settle in the body. As toxins, acids and slags, the pollutants are then deposited in the organs and joints and in fat and connective tissues. There they remain like a time-bomb waiting to go off at a suitable moment and cause gratuitous harm. This accumulation of pollutants upsets the natural balance of the body and impairs the regular functioning of the organism formerly intact. On the one hand the pollutants flood into the body faster than the body is able to excrete them, and on the other hand they hinder the absorption of nutrients. Organs are then no longer able to fulfill their tasks and are finally forced to capitulate in the face of overwhelming odds.

For this reason, detoxification of the body should begin with the whole, not the parts. A therapy specifically designed for one particular ailment can work only if the body has been thoroughly cleansed beforehand. If the body's powers have already been weakened by being overloaded with toxins, there can be no healing of body and soul. It may be possible to improve this or that symptom but not to achieve a cure, since toxins and slags are hindering the body's efforts.

Before any specific therapy is applied, the body must be encouraged to follow the path of healing of its own accord. Often, after careful cleansing of the body, there is no further need for specific therapy, as specific ailments are often due to a general load of toxins, so the body can heal itself as soon as these are eliminated. If the body is thoroughly cleansed, specific ailments often vanish into thin air in having no further basis. The body's natural processes of self-regulation are unleashed and work smoothly again.

Assisted detoxification

Our metabolism works like a factory without breaks. Every day, new nutrients are taken in, processed and stored then excreted when no longer needed. Thus waste matter also accumulates during digestion, and detoxification is a natural and essential part of the metabolism. It is an important process for maintaining good health, especially as our bodies are loaded with pollutants not only in the form of metabolic end products but also in the form of many environmental toxins, viruses and bacteria. Detoxification is therefore a necessary and natural bodily process, not an invention of naturopathy or a mysterious and elusive process.

Many school doctors say that detoxification of the body is unnecessary, as the body purifies itself. This is only partly true, as the human body is exposed to more and more pollution of the environment with heavy metals, toxins, chemicals of all kinds and radioactivity. There are also more additives in food and personal care products, while compensating factors such as a healthy diet, enough exercise and stress relief are widely neglected. Hardly anyone would question the worth of brushing your teeth every day or caring for your personal hygiene, but doubt is often cast on the much more important inner cleansing of the body.

Hence everyone knows the benefits of thorough dental care, but who knows about vital organs such as the liver, bowels and kidneys? Do you cleanse these as carefully and thoroughly as your teeth. If this question were posed to a room of people, most likely the only response would be a raising of the eyebrows or a shrug of the shoulders. Nonetheless, we go regularly to the hairdresser and the nail salon and care for our skin as our envelope with vials of unguents, face masks, creams and serums, so why do we treat our bodies so lackadaisically in stuffing them with unhealthy and harmful food? Is it due to carelessness, complacency, habit or lack of awareness?

It may be due to a combination of all these. It may also be due to the fact that if your hair or fingernails are neglected, the result is soon apparent, whereas our bodies are more secretive and tolerate our neglect too patiently for too long, till we no longer feel really on form or are downright ill. But we should treat our bodies like delicate plants, which if cherished will blossom and bear fruit and give us continual pleasure but if left in dingy corners will only wither away.

A non-toxic way of life

Healing always begins with insight and the will to turn over a new leaf. Already in antiquity, Hippocrates put this truth into words which have lost nothing of their force and validity: '**If you are unwilling to change your life, you can't be helped**!' If a doctor would dare say this today, his patients might stagger to their feet, wobble off and dwindle slowly into the distance and never be seen again. Indeed even the word patient, which in Latin alludes to patience and suffering, seems to imply that changes cannot be brought about but only accepted. You can only lean back stoically, while waiting for recovery in the near future.

Finally you go to the doctor, to hand the responsibility over to him. You are convinced that he will manage do the trick by ironing out the mistakes and sins of the past, the cause of the ailment. Often, he will do his best for the sake of being obliging and moving on to the next patient. He will take out a pad and pen and prescribe a medication, but the path of least resistance may lead only in a circle.

To reach a peak you may have to follow a steep and stony path, and the first step is the realization that your future lies in your own hands. Your doctor sees you only now and then and may know little about your past and your way of life. You have a much ampler sheaf of memories and hopes reaching back into the past and forward into the future, so why not take over his role? We all have latent and unbridled powers of healing. We need only acknowledge them and change our way of life leading into the future. We must toss old habits away like heavy overcoats hampering our movements and remind ourselves that we are the authors and actors of our dramas.

The aim is healing on all levels, harmony with ourselves and a state of physical and mental well being. But health is not only the absence of disease and suffering but also the presence of vitality and equanimity. Health means being at one with ourselves and the world, where there is neither too much nor too little on either side of our balance. There is neither too much or too little food and exercise. There is neither muddle nor monotony, bustle nor boredom. The hurdles are high but not too high and the aims are meaningful. There is neither frenzy nor apathy, aggression nor depression. There is joy and serenity, a lightness without fears and sorrows. This is not a Utopian vision but a state of being.

Healing is always holistic and about the whole person, the aim being a harmony of body, mind and soul. Not only our bodies but also our souls and spirits call for healing. Our spirits long to be stimulated and furthered, not dulled by gazing passively at the screen of a television every day or by surfing for hour after hour in the Internet. Our souls long for us to be at peace with ourselves and our fellow humans, not to be poisoned by continual competition and envy. May we quench the thirst of body, spirit and soul, sate their hunger and heal their maladies. Our serenity should not be a haven on the far horizon but as close to us as a parasol to its shade.

There is no royal road to healing. The paths are as different and varied as the people following them, but the aim is always to notice when we stray from the right path and to veer back. Self-knowledge is the first step towards improvement, but our natural instincts are always ready to point the way. The further we stray from a natural way of life, the sicker we become, in spite of all the achievements of modern medicine. The way back to nature is the way back to health, and every day we have chances to take it.

Holistic detoxification

As mentioned above, the body has various organs such as the liver, kidneys and intestines for its own detoxification. The separate organs are closely networked with each other and work together optimally as team players. This is why it is important that all organs be healthy and capable, for only their overall interaction lets the body be thoroughly cleansed and detoxified.

Instinctive detoxification

Detoxification is one of the most important forms of healing, if not the most important, for body and mind. Every chronic ailment is due to overloading the body with pollutants. The practice of detoxifying the body goes back a long way and may be as old as humanity itself. It is found in practically all cultures and religions, so an occasional cleansing of the body must be due to a natural instinct. This intuitive behavior can also be found among other animals, who instinctively fast and refuse food if they are ill or have eaten something unsuitable. This inherent protective mechanism ensures that animals detoxify and heal themselves.

Often animals eat certain plants for the sake of detoxification. Some roll round in the mud or rub against the branches of trees to get rid of pests like mosquitoes and lice, and these practices too are kinds of detoxification. But nowadays we have got used to behaving so unnaturally that some of us no longer heed our instinct to purify and detoxify the body. There is no longer a healthy respect for the body's needs, and instinctive guidance is blandly ignored as being at odds with modern life. It is time to pay attention to the body's sound advice and to act on it.

A toxic overflow

A chronically poisoned body is like an overflowing waste-bin. Basically the body purifies itself, as we have seen, and its purification system is made up of a sophisticated array of interconnected detoxification processes which many organs are involved in. This sophisticated means of detoxification can truly be called a masterpiece of creation or evolution, so why should a helping hand be needed if the body is already self-sufficient and competent?

Well, certainly the body is busily detoxifying itself, day in and day out, to rebuff or to render harmless many materials, but we are no longer in our natural surroundings. We are exposed to countless pollutants, many of which mercilessly find their way into the lungs, the gut or skin then penetrate more deeply into the body. Even people fully aware of the problem and keen to avoid pollutants are nonetheless often exposed and vulnerable.

In offices or workshops for instance, we are exposed to plastics and paints in forms including furniture, carpeting and wall paints, and on eating junk food in the lunch hour, we take in many harmful additives. Those of us who work out of doors on the land are contaminated with herbicides and insecticides, so the problem is so pervasive that a change in our way of life or even a change of scene is only a partial solution. We have to pay attention to not only what we eat but also other things around us like our cosmetics and clothes and how we clean them.

It should also be noted that many pollutants affecting us today have existed only in the wake of modern organic chemistry and its arsenal of pesticides, herbicides, insecticides and innumerable detergents. The situation is not improved by additives in food and cosmetics or by certain substances in furniture, building materials and clothing, not to mention radioactivity, drug residues in animal foods and chemicals in the amalgam of dental fillings. Thus we are confronted by pollutants in every sector of our lives, often without even being aware of it. We also eat too much and move too little.

Stress and few chances to relax affect the body too. On the whole we do too much bad and too little good to our bodies. This leads to its being gradually overloaded and poisoned, and at some point event the best detoxification processes are exhausted and cannot wholly fulfill their tasks. The body slowly loses its balance and is unable to regain it. Being unable to remove enough toxins, it is forced to store them for the time being, and mostly they are stored in the connective tissues. This is because these tissues are connected to all organs, not only to the lymphatic system, blood vessels and cells of the nervous system.

The need for temporarily storage is due to the fact that the waste, made of up slag, toxins and acids, is otherwise in the way and prevents regular detoxification. By dumping it in the connective tissues, the body is able to keep on functioning, more or less, for the time being, but the price paid may include an orange discoloration of the skin, harm to connective tissues and problems with the veins.

If the harmful materials are not gradually removed from the connective tissue or if even more waste accumulates, the capacity of the connective tissues is no longer enough. Harmful materials from the whole body can no longer be taken up and later discharged. The barrel is then full to overflowing, a sign that many chronic ailments are bound to follow.

Just imagine what would happen if garbage were collected not once a week but once a month. It would spill all over the streets throughout the township. The whole place would stink and be overrun by vermin, parasites, bacteria and viruses. It would hardly be possible to stay healthy. The same is true of the township of your body. It becomes a slum, where toxins spread as surely as an epidemic. This shows how practical it is to deal with the waste promptly through regular detoxification. Neglect may otherwise change you, but not for the better.

Helping the body to cope

The organs in general should be helped in their efforts to remove toxins, then they will remove them more effectively. They should also be protected and regenerated by suitable means, for if cared for properly, they will stay healthy and work well. Moreover, the body as a whole should be detoxified.

The harmful materials stored in the body should be eliminated, but for the sake of avoiding symptoms of acute poisoning, this should be done slowly and prudently. If all poisons were **released at once** from the connective tissues, the whole body could be acutely affected. But of course this is no reason to leave them there indefinitely like mines in a rice field.

As we have seen, the toxins in the connective tissues do no direct harm at first, but at some point they fill the waste-bins to overflowing. This is extremely risky, as they suddenly contaminate the whole body. A slow but sustained detoxification may serve to avoid this fiasco.

To begin with, a further intake of toxins should be hindered. Harmful chemicals such as nicotine and alcohol should ideally be avoided, to let the body be optimally detoxified and cleansed. The body should also be freed from any kind of stress, to let it calm down and deal mainly with the necessary healing processes. You can thereby come back to yourself and regain your inner balance.

Common toxins

If the body is a chronic victim of poisoning, there are many possible suspects, listed below:

Processes of decay and fermentation within the body
Degradation products of the metabolism
Acidosis
Pathogens, like bacteria, viruses and fungi
Chemicals in textiles, food, furniture and cosmetics
Solvents, like acetone
Dyes
Softeners
Heavy metals, like mercury, lead and calcium
Fibers, like asbestos and glass wool
Insecticides, fungicides and herbicides
Manure as a 'natural' fertilizer
Mold toxins
Drugs used in medicine

Drugs used in chemotherapy
Exposure to radiation
Recreational drugs, like alcohol and nicotine
Too little or too much food
Sugar, white flour and too much animal protein
Food additives, like preservatives, antioxidants, stabilizers, emulsifiers, colorants, flavorings, flavor enhancers, pickling salts, sweeteners and sugar substitutes
Heavy metals in food, like aluminum in lye pastry, mercury in fish, copper as a stabilizer for chlorophyll, which serves as a green colorant in liqueurs and sweets for instance
Residues of antibiotics and hormones in meat
Residues of insecticides and pesticides in fruits and greens
Contaminated air (ozone)
Scars
Cramped and tense postures
Anxiety and depression
A lack of refreshing sleep
A lack of exercise, especially in the open air
Stress
Noise
Deadlines to meet and quality to keep

Chronic poisoning of the body overloads the organs of purification like the liver, kidneys, gut, lungs, lymph system and skin. If they are continually overloaded, the pollutants are redirected, which may lead to fever, eczema, diarrhea and acne. Overloading the body with pollutants and toxins also leads to the deposition of metabolic waste. Cell walls then thicken, disrupting the supply of nutrients to the cells and changing the milieu of cells and tissues. It also affects the circulation of the blood, as blood cells become less elastic and more rigid. In general, the body becomes acidified, so persistently poising the body creates a vicious circle with far-reaching consequences. Breaking it is a precondition for all detoxification measures.

Chronic poisoning

Harmful substances in food

Keen to produce foods even more cost-effectively and efficiently, many food manufacturers are eager to use pesticides, herbicides, fungicides and a whole range of other harmful substances. Also the wish of many customers to eat highly processed and visually appealing food encourages the producers to rely on using more and more additives. Certain pollutants and poisons occur naturally in some foods so can be avoided only by eating the foods less or not at all.

To avoid additives, you can carefully prepare the food yourself from unadulterated biological sources if possible. Fruit and vegetables in particular are not as good for the health if treated with pesticides, herbicides or fungicides. Heavy metals too are found in conventionally grown vegetables, like cadmium in spinach, and genetically modified fruit and vegetables with still unclear effects on the human body should ideally be avoided.

Meat often contains antibiotics and hormones, so if you are loath to stop eating meat, you should at least ensure that the animals have been kept under natural conditions. Even meat from wild animals such as stags, deer and boar may not be free from radioactivity, and the same is true of forest mushrooms such as chanterelles. Grilling meat produces polycyclic aromatic hydrocarbons (PAHs), which increase the risk of colorectal cancer. It is especially risky to eat red meat from cattle, calves, pigs, goats or sheep. Cured meats and sausages are pickled with nitrite, a cause of cancer of the stomach and esophagus.

Phosphate, added for instance to sausages, meat and processed cheese, may ruin kidneys already harmed and also trigger cardiovascular diseases. Fish meals are healthy, but long-lived predatory fish like tuna, swordfish, monkfish, sharks and eels may contain notable amounts of mercury, as it accumulates in the food chain. Some shells and kinds of fish such as soused herring contain arsenic. Eggs too may contain arsenic if the hens have been fed fish-meal. Feeding fish-meal to hens I banned in the European Union, but the feeding is seldom checked. Arsenic is still found in rice from Asia, as arsenic locked in the soil is more available in flooded fields.

Highly toxic molds (aflatoxins) are often found in pistachios, peanuts, coffee, cereals and bread, whereas aluminum may pass from food cans into the food and is often excessively present in lye biscuits. Bitter almonds contain hydrocyanic acid, so eighteen are often enough to kill a normal grown up. In recent years, acrylamide has gained a certain notoriety. This carcinogenic substance is produced if starchy foods such as chips or fried potatoes are baked, roasted or deeply fried or if crunchy cereals or cereal cakes are heated or baked. Moreover, many foods now contain colorants, flavor enhancers, preservatives and artificial flavors, so there are hardly any foods left without harmful or toxic ingredients.

Pollutants in textiles

Not only food but also textiles contain a whole range of pollutants and toxins. But since we do not ingest clothes but only wear them on the outsides of our bodies, the problem of highly contaminated clothing is not so obvious. Nonetheless our skin is able to absorb chemicals too, so pollutants in clothes are absorbed in high concentrations. Unfortunately, clothes are viewed as being only commodities, so their toxic contents are hardly checked, especially in Asia, where the rules and regulations are even laxer. Unknown to its owner, a wardrobe is often full of harmful fabrics, but this problem can be avoided only by wearing clothes with ecological certificates or by wearing the same clothes for year after year, whatever the changes in fashion. We can move on without listing and examining all the pollutants and toxins.

Death in the living room

Toxins in homes and workplaces are poisons, mostly organic, which may be present in building materials, floor coverings or furniture. They may be in the building materials themselves in the form of paints, varnishes, carpets or PVC floor coverings or may be introduced into the rooms over time, for instance as wood preservatives. Some living rooms have been found to contain a cocktail of as many as 700 000 different chemicals, which is a really frightening figure, as we spend much or most of our time indoors, be it at work or at home. Moreover, most organic compounds have only a low vapor pressure, so they are released slowly over decades.

What is worrying is also the accumulation of organic compounds, as these are very soluble in lipids, so they accumulate in the food chain and adipose tissues. They are not always acutely toxic to humans, but their chronic effects such as a puzzling fatigue and lack of motivation are all the more devastating. Moreover, the specific cause is often hard to pinpoint. What can be done? Basically, rooms should always be well aired, and we should go out into the open every day. Especially in old buildings, like those with wooden panels overhead and wooden floors, it is useful to let living rooms be inspected by a responsible institute or to send the institute suitable samples. When buying furniture or other necessities, you may heed eco-labels like the 'blue angel'.

Formaldeyhyde, PCP, PCB, DDT, mold, polystyrene, asbestos, dust mites and solvents are among the most harmful and common poisons in living rooms. Formaldehyde is nonetheless widely used, even today, as a disinfectant, preservative and binder of synthetic resins and is also used to make clothing less likely to wrinkle and crease. It can be found in many other common items like leather, cosmetics, detergents, softeners, wallpapers, carpets, furniture, paints, adhesives and varnishes. It is even applied to sheets of paper, newspapers and books, though it is known to induce cancer.

In Germany, PCP (pentachlorphenol) was used to preserve wood till the 1980s then banned, though it is still in some old furniture and imported chipboards, rugs, carpets and other textiles. In New Zealand, it was used to preserve wood till 1988 and was sold by Shell in the form of a watery solution to kill moss; in the United States, it was sold till the early 1980s but is now used only on utility poles and railroad sleepers; and in Chile, it was used till the early 1990s as a fungicide, to reduce the 'blue stains' in pinewood. In 2015, countries which had signed the Stockholm Convention agreed to ban it. PCP also induces cancer and is often contaminated with dioxin.

Carbolineum is made up of various higher boiling anthracene oils derived from coal tar. It is still approved for outdoor use as a wood preservative, in being effective against bacteria and rot, but there are still many other items with residues of carbolineum, though it too induces cancer.

Asbestos has already achieved infamy. It is made of of fibrous silicate mineral fibers, which are not only strong but also resistant to acid and heat and are thus useful as insulation. Hence it was widely used in the building industry for roofing, outer walls and floors, till it was banned. This occurred in Germany in 1993 and even earlier in the United States, where the Environmental Protection Agency ordered it to be phased out in 1989. Unfortunately industrial producers then challenged the ruling, which left many loopholes for them to exploit, though Washington State banned the use of asbestos in the brakes of vehicles in 2010.

Asbestos is still common in Vietnam, where according to a study of three hundred families in

Yen Bai and Than Hóa, 85% of the households have roofs of asbestos sheets and only 5% of the residents have learned of its harmful effects. In Britain blue, brown and white asbestos were all banned by 1999, though some is still present in factories and offices, whose owners have to ensure that none deteriorates.

In Australia it was banned from building products in 1989 and cannot be imported, used or recycled. In New Zealand it was banned in 2015, except for a few exceptions to be reviewed on a case-by-case basis. In Japan it was banned in 2006, in South Korea in 2009 and in Canada in 2018, except for use in military and nuclear facilities. In most developed countries, asbestos is dumped as hazardous waste in landfill sites.

Mold is the greatest inducer of cancer, but spores are inhaled in moldy homes. Its presence may be due to faults in building materials, to the closeness of furniture to walls and to not enough airing of rooms.

Styrene is an unsaturated, aromatic hydrocarbon, which serves as a monomer for the further processing of plastics like polystyrene and is classified as harmful.

PCBs (polychlorinated biphenyls) have been used as capacitors in washing-machines and as plasticizers in paints, plastics, sealants and insulating materials. Their chlorine compounds are toxic and cause cancer and belong to the so-called dirty dozen of organic toxins banned globally by the Stockholm Convention in 2001, but PCBs can still be found in the ground, in water and elsewhere.

DDT is another of the dirty dozen, though it was widely used till the 1980s inf wood preservatives, owing to its effectiveness as an insecticide. It may now be used only to kill insects which otherwise spread malaria.

Chronic poisoning by amalgam

For many decades, amalgam was the material most commonly used for tooth fillings, but toxic mercury is released on their removal. Even if they remain in the mouth, small amounts of mercury are continually released, especially if fillings become porous in the course of time. The discomfort caused by amalgam fillings, even after removal, is often tedious and non-specific. Typical symptoms include chronic fatigue, exhaustion, lack of drive and difficulty in concentrating, so old amalgam fillings should be replaced if possible by more suitable and less harmful alternatives.

To avoid harm from the leaking of mercury during the removal of fillings, a dentist should always take preemptive measures. The room should be well aired, and medical carbon may be used before and after removal, to absorb any amalgam released. A special clean up with the help of vacuum suction may serve to remove any mercury leaking. Generally, as little drilling should be done as possible and the pieces of amalgam be removed intact.

Apart from the teeth to be treated, the inside of the mouth should also be covered with rubber dam, a kind of rubbery cloth. During the removal of mercury, overheating may be avoided by working slowly, which lessens the amount of mercury released. Inhalation of mercury may be avoided by using an oxygen nasogastric tube or an oxygen mask, and eyes must be protected by wearing goggles.

After removal of the fillings, sodium thiosulfate is used to bind and compound the amalgam. No more than two or three fillings should be removed per session, and there should be adequate intervals between sessions. After the removal, it is useful to undergo detoxification with a high dose of vitamin C, along with calcium, a vitamin B complex and vitamin E. Detoxification is also helped by ingesting blue and green algae.

Paths of detoxification

The body has various organs of detoxification as well as numerous regulatory mechanisms responsible for its cleansing and detoxification. In the course of metabolic activity in general, these natural pathways of detoxification free the body from slags, acids and toxins. But this is done not only by organs but also by cells, each of which has its own metabolism and means of waste-disposal and detoxification. The main organs responsible for detoxification and purification are:

liver
gut
kidneys
skin
lymphatic system
lungs

The lymphatic system is not a single organ but a body-wide network of lymphatic organs and vessels, to be looked at more closely later.

Liver

The liver works for us day and night. Countless processes involved in the metabolism occur in it, so it is sometimes called the powerhouse of the body. As the central organ in the metabolism it has a huge range of responsibilities. It has to control the balance of energy and hormones, the processing and storage of fats, proteins and carbohydrates, the production of vital proteins like coagulation factors, and the production of bile. It also helps to establish a balance between acids and alkalies and converts some substances soluble in fat into substances soluble in water, letting them pass out of the body in urine.

But above all, the liver is our foremost organ of decontamination. All poisons which enter us through the skin, the gut or the lungs pass through the liver. It is tirelessly involved in modifying toxins, to let them be eliminated through the kidneys or the gut, so it is the first address for the detoxification of alien substances like alcohol, chemicals, bacteria and viruses.

Moreover, the liver breaks the body's own substances down. These include hormones no longer needed, faulty cells, decrepit red blood cells and waste products of the protein mechanism. In removing bacteria from the gut, it also supports the immune system. It eliminates substances like bilirubin, cholesterol, metabolic products and medications through bile, till they are passed out in the faeces.

Gut

The gut is crucial in the excretion of toxins and metabolic end products. For instance it takes water from unusable food remains, letting them be excreted in faeces. These are made up of water, the food remains, cells shed by the gut's mucous membrane, secretions of the digestive gland, gut bacteria and products of fermentation and decay. A healthy gut flora and a regulated digestion are key preconditions for a smooth detoxification of the gut, which is also important for protecting the immune system. In fact 80% of the cells of the immune system are found in the gut's mucous membrane.

The gut's flora also serves as an important barrier preventing poisons and pathogens from entering the rest of the body. Keeping the gut healthy and functional is essential for detoxification. Its functioning depends on many factors, not only on a healthy flora but also on a balanced diet, on a good blood circulation in the gut, on a proper absorption of nutrients by the gut's villi, on how long food lingers in the gut and on the gut's peristalsis.

Kidneys

The kidneys too are continually working at top speed, letting metabolic end products be passed out in urine several times a day. Blood flows continuously from all parts of the body through the kidneys, to let soluble toxins and pollutants be removed. Every day, the kidneys filter and cleanse up to 1 500 liters of blood, and the filtrate is passed out in about 1.5 liters of urine. Among other things, nitrogen-containing decomposition products such as urea from food rich in proteins are passed out, while substances good for the body such as minerals are reabsorbed. But these processes can work only if the person drinks enough liquid to flush the pollutants out, as water increases the blood's volume, making the work easier.

The kidneys also play a key role in regulating the balance of acids and alkalies in the body. They deal with an excess of acid in several sophisticated ways. If for instance they are swamped by acids, they eliminate fewer alkalies, to restore the balance. At the same time, they increasingly replace acids in the form of hydrogen ions with sodium and potassium ions, while organic acids and acidic nitrogen compounds pass into urine, which is then stored in the bladder till excreted. Hence it is possible to stimulate the kidneys, to encourage them to get rid of more acids.

Skin

With a surface area of up to two square meters, the skin is our biggest organ. Its range of tasks is proportionate to its size, as it has to protect us from heat, cold and radiation, to shield the inner organs from pressure and shock and to prevent pathogens from finding their way into the body. Glands in the lower layers of the skin produce sweat, which coats it protectively, but if the body is too acidified or contaminated, the glands produce more sweat, to get rid of more pollutants and acids and to thicken the protective layer.

Sweating – whether in sport or a sauna – is thereby healthy and restores the body's acid-alkali balance. Last but not least, the term 'healthily sweating' is also applied to people with colds or influenza, when more sweat gets rid of more microbes. The glands also act as a filter for pathogens, acids and toxins like mercury, which are then sweated out, as long as blood circulates well in the skin.

There are various ways to cause healthy sweating. For instance, physical activity and the associated contractions of muscles stimulate circulation of the blood, so in just an hour of physical activity, we may secrete half a liter of sweat. A massage or the heat of a sauna or unusually warm bath likewise causes vessels to dilate and promote healthy sweating and thus to get rid of pollutants. Under normal conditions, we lose between 1 and 1.5 liters of sweat a day, though it evaporates so fast that we hardly notice. All in all, sweating is natural, though a lot of sweat may be a sign of serious illness or a greater need for detoxification, and a little sweat like only 0.5 liters a day may be due to spending a lot of time in sitting.

Lymphatic system

This is responsible for instance for cleansing and detoxifying the body's water and for keeping it clear. It collects bacteria, bacterial toxins, viruses, fungi, heavy metals, chemicals, cell debris and defunct or dysfunctional cells, which float in the lymph till reaching the lymph nodes, where they are filtered out. In the lymph nodes, pathogens are destroyed, toxins neutralized and bacteria eliminated. Many lymph nodes are found in the groin, neck and armpits and have lymphocytes and phagocytes able to kill cancer cells. If the lymphatic system has too much to cope with, unclean lymph may enter the blood and poison the whole organism, so the lymph should be cleansed regularly and its activity be stimulated.

Lungs

The lungs are where oxygen is exchanged. Oxygen is breathed in together with air then is removed by blood passing through the lungs. This replaces it with carbon dioxide, which in being acidic has to be removed from the body. On account of stress, tension, sloth or habit, our breathing is often too shallow, so stress reduction and physical exercise play a key role in improvement. Someone at rest breathes in about half a liter of air with each breath, whereas an athlete may breath in ten to twelve times as much at the moment of greatest physical exertion. The greater the exertion, the more oxygen we need and breathe in.

If the body is supplied with too little oxygen, it may become acidified. We may then react instinctively by breathing out more forcefully, as this is the right way to get rid of more carbon dioxide and potential acid. The lungs thereby take over the responsibility of oxidizing the acids and eliminating them by breathing out. Gaseous toxins such as acetone as well as putrefactive gases containing nitrogen or sulfur can likewise be released through the lungs. Deep breathing increases the rate of this purification, so our breathing can usefully be improved by hour-long sports like walking, running, cycling, swimming and gymnastics.

Cleansing by the system

While cleansing the colon or detoxifying the liver is often a priority of any detoxification therapy, detoxification of the lymphatic system is often neglected. This may be due to the fact that the system works discretely behind the scenes so seldom attracts attention. Its role in detoxification is nonetheless huge, as if removes and neutralizes pollutants isolated from the body's own defense cells (proteins, cell debris, toxins, other pollutants, bacteria and viruses, and cancer cells) and excretes them.

The lymphatic system can properly be called the body's purification system, so if it is unable to work well, the body is flooded with slag, toxins, bacteria, viruses, fungi, cell debris and faulty cells. It goes without saying that this may lead to a whole range of ailments, so a holistic cleansing of the lymphatic system is an important way to prevent or cure ailments of all kinds. This keeps the body's water wonderfully clean and healthy.

The lymphatic system must be credited with not shying away from dealing with the roughest and toughest waste. The lymph capillaries absorb bacteria, bacterial toxins, viruses, fungi, heavy metals, chemicals, cell debris, dysfunctional and degenerate cells and bear them to the lymph nodes. These work as filters and detoxification centers for the whole system, removing and neutralizing all kinds of pollutants, till the purified lymph is allowed to seep into the bloodstream.

All in all, it is hardly surprising that our health crucially depends on the performance of the lymphatic system, since the lymph nodes are the police and guardians of our health. Packed with phagocytes and lymphocytes, they kill bacteria and literally feed on cancer cells but, given such a range of responsibilities, they are sometimes overloaded with all kinds of waste like toxins, fats, bacteria, viruses, parasites, fungi, slime, mucilage and flawed cells. If this happens often and the lymphatic activity is not stimulated enough, the nodes' efficiency or that of the defensive cells within them is bound to be affected.

The lymph may then slow down and finally stagnate, like standing water into which poison is continually seeping. The water no longer flows off, so the poison accumulates and the water is unable to support life. The image is drastic but fitting. If the lymphatic system is overloaded, poisons and slag from the lymph may enter the bloodstream and slowly but surely poison the body.

A blockage of flow may cause discomfort like swollen eyes, thick legs and hands, and cellulitis. There may be a leaden and puzzling fatigue, a loss of performance and focus, a chronic headache, inflammation of the sinuses, a sore throat, colds, acne and menstrual cramps. In the long run, chronic diseases may become acute and lead for instance to cancer. The lymphatic system is not only responsible for detoxification but, along with the gut, is also the main part of our immune system, so the need for holistically caring for it can hardly be overestimated.

The lymphatic system has a certain feature which makes regular detoxification even more important. Its vessels run parallel to and next to those of the blood, but whereas the blood is continually pumped by the heart, the lymph is left to flow of its own accord, so a thorough cleansing of the lymphatic system has two main aims:

Aims of lymphatic cleansing

The main aims are:

Stimulation and activation of the lymphatic flow, to ensure that pathogens, cancer cells and poisons are flushed out of the body quickly and effectively.

Relief and cleansing of the liver, gut and kidneys as other organs of purification, so let them cope without relying on the lymph. The lymphatic system can then devote more time to regenerating itself.

Cleansing the gut first

Due to the close connection between the lymphatic system and the gut, any measures taken to purify the former should also include measures to improve the gut flora. If there are many toxins, slag and pollutants in the gut, the gut passes some on to the lymph and impedes its flow, so a good probiotic should be taken in the course of lymphatic cleansing. This lets the gut's mucous membranes regenerate and rids them of putrefactive bacteria and fungi for instance. It also strengthens the gut's immune system and function of purification.

The lymphatic system

In the body, materials and fluids are exchanged by blood vessels and extracellular space. This space is where dross accumulates, which would otherwise overload the blood. The dross includes harmful materials and big molecules, which the lymphatic system takes up and bears away.

The lymphatic system keeps the body's water clean, healthy and clear so is responsible for cleansing and detoxification. In the lymph flowing through its vessels, there are bacteria, heavy metals, cell debris, bacterial toxins, chemicals, viruses, fungi and flawed or decrepit cells. These are filtered out by the lymph nodes, which are especially numerous in the groin, neck and armpits. In them pathogens and toxins are destroyed, poisons neutralized, bacteria eliminated and cancer cells eaten by phagocytes.

Along with the bloodstream, the lymphatic system is the body's main circulation and transport system. It differs from the bloodstream in having no central pump and is made up of lymph channels, nodes and fluid. These are part of its one-way system, whose main function is to return lymph from the outskirts of the body to the bloodstream.

Throughout the body, the lymphatic system runs next to the blood system for the sake of interaction. Fluid for instance passes from blood vessels into tissues then from there into lymphatic vessels with other important tasks. The lymph bears not only excess water but also various nutrients. In particular, it bears big molecules unable to pass through capillary walls into the blood. These include molecules of fats (lipids) and proteins.

The lymphatic vessels also supply cells with nutrients, and what is useless to the cells remains in the vessels, but the lymph not only brings food but also removes waste products of the metabolism. These include cell debris, pathogens and toxins, which are born away to the lymph nodes, to be dealt with there. The lymphatic system is thus am important part of the immune system, involved in detoxifying the body. The intruders are confronted by lymphocytes, which react to them by swiftly multiplying. The remains of destroyed pathogens and cell debris are then released into venous blood and finally passed out through the kidneys.

The system's tasks

Drainage: the removal of fluids, proteins, cell debris, poisons and pathogens from the intercellular space.

Immune function: lymphocytes circulating in the lymph vessels eat all kinds of pathogens, which is why there are many lymphatic structures like the lymph nodes and tonsils in and around the throat, where pathogens of all kinds are most likely to enter the body. The lymphatic organs also play a key role in the immune function of the lymph system (see the chapter *Lymphatic organs*).

Detoxification: the lymph channels bear all kinds of waste to the lymph nodes, where the lymph is detoxified.

Transportation: some materials such as fats cannot be borne through the blood system on account of their size, so their molecules are borne by the lymph.

Lymph

In his novel *The Magic Mountain*, Thomas Mann alludes to the lymph as *the juice of juices*. Why the lymph is such an important juice, what the lymph nodes and lymphocytes are and what happens when the system becomes muddled will now be explained.

The lymph (Latin: *lympha*, clear water) is the fluid in the body's lymphatic vessels, and its hue varies from part to part of the body. In the extremities is is clear and colorless but around the belly, it is milky white or yellowish due to tiny particles of fat absorbed from the stomach and gut. This variety is known as *chyle*. Resembling both tissue fluid (intercellular fluid) and blood plasma, lymph is squeezed out of blood vessels and is made up of shaped materials (cells) and plasma. It has a pH of 7.41, is initially like tissue fluid and has a so-called water-load (cell debris, pathogens and other pollutants), fat-load and protein-load.

Composition of the lymph

Water
Calcium
Potassium
Sodium
Glucose
Creatine
Urea
Phosphate
White blood cells
Fats
Protein
Enzymes of various kinds (amylases, catalases, dipeptidases and lipases)
Fibrinogen and fibrin-precursors

Fibrinogen and fibrin are responsible for coagulation in stagnant lymph. The lymph also contains on average two to six grams of egg-white (proteins) per liter, depending on the part of the body. After a fatty meal, there may be as much as one or two grams of lipids (fats) per liter, owing to which it looks milky and is called *chyle*, after *chylos*, Greek for juice. The lymph transports solutes like proteins and lipids as well as waste.

Formation of the lymph

The lymph comes from extra-capillary fluid, as during circulation a part of the blood plasma is constantly squeezed into intercellular spaces in the surrounding tissues. These are washed and saturated by the plasma, so lymph is basically derived from fluid in blood vessels. This serves to supply the surrounding cells with nutrients as well as to remove metabolic products and other waste. Later about 90% of the tissue fluid returns to the blood vessels, and the fluid remaining collects as lymph in the lymph vessels.

Every day the body produces more than five liters of milky and watery lymph, which flows through its own system of vessels. There it is reduced to about two liters and reintroduced through the left subclavian vein into the bloodstream. Compared to the venous system for the blood, the system for the lymph has a low transport capacity of two to four liters a day, so it disposes of only about 10% of the amount of fluid squeezed into the tissues.

Before being passed back into the blood, the lymph is filtered by numerous lymph nodes. Humans have about 600, many of them in the armpits, neck, groins, elbows and knees. The nodes are also an important part of the immune system, as pathogens are drawn to them from diseased parts of the body, to be isolated, identified and destroyed by dendritic cells.

The greater the number of pathogens in the body, the greater the number of antibodies are made as antidotes, to drive these aliens out of the body. As a result, the lymph nodes may visibly swell and hurt, though this is only a sign that they are working overtime. Nonetheless, if the lymphatic drainage is hindered, there may be congestion, revealed by symptoms of poisoning, more frequent ailments, lymphoma or inflammation of the lymphatic vessels.

Lymph nodes

Also called lymph glands, these are filters for cleansing the lymph. This continually brings to them pathogens, poisons and cell debris, which are there rendered harmless by macrophages and lymphocytes. The lymph nodes are especially suited to this task in being the place where lymphocytes are produced. Most lymphocytes then remain in the lymphatic system and only a few enter the bloodstream.

Lymph nodes are found throughout the body except in the central nervous system, and most of them are in clusters. Altogether the human body has about 600 of them, the best known being in the neck, armpits and groin, where they collect waste and pathogens from the neck, head and limbs. The bean-shaped nodes are five to twenty millimeters across and encapsulated in tissues like connective tissues. Each capsule contains an outer cortex and inner medulla.

The lymph nodes are where lymph is collected and filtered, then the filtrate can leave the nodes through laxative vessels (Latin: *vasa efferentia*). The lymph nodes are used mainly for detoxification but also for immune defense. They are where incoming lymph is checked for harmful materials and pathogens, then any present trigger the process of detoxification off. Lymphocytes swiftly multiply and destroy all unwanted intruders.

Their multiplication causes the lymph nodes to swell, as may be seen during throat infections, colds and influenza, around the throat, lower jaw and nape, whereas during Pfeiffer's glandular fever, nodes may swell in the throat, armpits, nape and/or groin. In the case of malignant tumors or certain serious ailments such as HIV or syphilis, lymph nodes may swell throughout the body. The lymphocytes made in the nodes are not confined to them. Those matching a certain kind of germ are sent as immune cells through the body, to deal with the infection on location, but lymphocytes and phagocytes are most numerous and closely packed in the nodes, so once the lymph has been filtered and concentrated there, it contains only immune cells and protein.

The system's structure & purpose

The lymphatic system (Latin: *Systema lymphaticum*) denotes all the lymph channels in the body as well as the lymphatic organs which the lymph nodes belong to. It also includes the spleen, the thymus and the lymphatic tissues in the digestive tract like the Peyer plaques in the small intestine and throat (throat, tongue and tonsils).

The lymphatic system is an important part of the immune system for combating pathogens, foreign bodies and pathologically changed parts of the body like tumor cells. It is used for not only detoxification and defense but also for transporting various molecules (see the chapter *Lymph*) and it interacts closely with the bloodstream. It is not a single organ but a system of organs spread throughout the body.

The system's organs

The lymphatic organs are specialized for the differentiation and multiplication of lymphocytes and consist of primary and secondary organs.

Primary lymphatic organs

Thymus
Bone marrow

The primary lymphatic organs are the places where precursor cells differentiate into immuno-competent T and B lymphocytes.

Secondary lymphatic organs

Lymph follicle
Peyer's patches
Tonsils
Spleen
Lymph nodes
Worm-shaped appendix

In the secondary lymphatic organs, a specific immune reaction is triggered by a meeting of antigens and immunocompetent lymphocytes.

Lymphocytes

The lymph contains lymphocytes, very important for the immune system. Lymphocytes belong to the group of white blood cells (leukocytes) and are the smallest of these but also the main bearers of targeted immune defense. They make up about 25 –

40% of white cells in the blood. The group of lymphocytes includes the B lymphocytes, the T lymphocytes and the natural killer cells (NK cells).

The main tasks of lymphocytes are to recognize and remove foreign bodies from the organism. Lymphocytes are molded by foreign materials and belong to the adaptive (acquired) immune system, so they need more time to react to pathogens, but the acquired defense is then more effective than the innate defense.

B-lymphocytes (B cells)

These are made in the bone marrow and are part of the so-called acquired immune defense. The *B* stands for Bursa fabrici, which is a lymphatic organ producing lymphocytes in birds, but the *B* is now often associated with bone marrow. After being made in the bone marrow, the mature B lymphocytes circulate in the lymphatic system and in the bloodstream. In being the only cells able to make antibodies, B-lymphocytes can truly be called our main bodyguards in the fight against viruses, bacteria and fungi.

B cells use their B-receptors to recognize certain foreign structures. The receptors then grip the alien antigens and bind them, but binding them in itself is not enough. Purpose-made antibodies are likewise needed to destroy the antigens, so B-lymphocytes migrate to the nearest lymph-node, where antibodies begin to form. Later, a few of the B-lymphocytes change into B-memory-cells, which keep on circulating in the blood even after the end of the infection. If the same kind of antigen reinfects the body later, its contact with a B-memory-cell leads to a much faster reaction, as the cell can remember it at once.

The use of B-lymphocytes in defense is also called humoral immunity, which alludes to interaction between the antigen and antibody.

T-lymphocytes

Also known as T-cells, these are likewise formed in the bone marrow but then migrate to the thymus (hence the name T-lymphocytes), where they mature. Various kinds of T-lymphocytes are then formed, to deal with tallying tasks. T-cells recognize foreign materials so they continually and rigorously check the blood for their presence. Through the blood and lymphatic tissue, they spread all through the body, checking cells for any pathological changes.

Unlike B-lymphocytes, T-lymphocytes produce no antibodies but attach themselves without any intermediate steps to cells affected by pathogens and also produce defensive substances. T-lymphocytes live a long time and remember any pathogens which have found their way into the body, so if the body is reinfected, they react fast and effectively.

Natural killer cells

NK-cells have the task of recognizing and directly destroying abnormal cells such as infected cells or cancer cells. This is called programmed cell death (apoptosis), initiated by the natural killer cells. These have no receptors specific to certain antigens so belong to the innate immune system. Like other lymphocytes, natural killer cells develop from lymphatic progenitor cells in the bone marrow and later migrate to the bloodstream. They are bigger than T-lymphocytes and B-lymphocytes.

Disclaimer

As regards the presentation below, the reader may rest assured that the author has taken great care to ensure that statements made in this book are scientifically up to date. But findings in the domains of medicine and pharmacy are never final but are subject to an ongoing process of development. Information can be based only on the state of knowledge at the time of the book's publication, so the author can accept no responsibility for later discrepancies.

The reader heeds the advice offered in this book at his or her own risk. The author accepts no liability for injury to a person, harm to property, or loss of money due to heeding any of the advice.

As regards the indicated and recommended dosages for the medicines mentioned and food supplements – be they herbal, biochemical, homeopathic or other – the reader may rest assured that the author has taken great care to ensure that they too are scientifically up to date. Nonetheless, she can accept no liability for suggested doses. Each dose is taken at the reader's own risk.

The author has no relationship with manufacturers of medicines or food supplements and obtains no financial benefit from mentioning any of these.

Now, let us clarify how to keep the lymphatic system healthy. The following measures will ensure that the lymph is kept clean and flowing.

Sustaining the lymph's flow

Drink enough or about 2.5 liters a day, preferably non-fizzy water, fruit tea and herbal tea or diluted juices. In summer, when exercising or sweating, our need for fluid may increase. The fact that our bodies have twice as much lymph as blood shows how greatly the lymph needs fluid. The more watery the lymph is, the more easily it can flow and fulfill its function of detoxification, whereas if too little is drunk, the lymph thickens and becomes viscous and may even stagnate.

If it becomes viscous, harmful toxins, bacteria, slag and cancerous cells remain in the body, and the likelier it is that ailments will develop. Only if enough fluid is absorbed can the lymph be cleansed and only then can other detoxification measures be effective. If enough water is drunk, the liver and kidneys are better rinsed with blood and can more effectively fulfill their function of detoxification.

Stimulating the system

For the lymph to be properly set in motion, there is a need for enough exercise. Unlike the bloodstream with its heart, the lymphatic system has no pump, so it has to be actively stimulated for the fluid to move on. This can be done for instance by breathing deeply into the belly and by physical exercise such as swimming, hiking, dancing, cycling or even leisurely strolling. This ensures that the lymph moves on and that the lymphatic system remains fit. The circulation of the lymph depends on the pressure in the tissues, the muscles, the walls of the lymphatic vessels and on the movement of the whole system of muscles.

Movement creates pressure in the tissues and thereby drives the lymph forwards, and muscular activity helps the lymph to flow by causing the lymphatic vessels between the muscles to be pushed together rhythmically, which effectively pumps the lymph upwards.

Besides moving around every day, you you treat yourself to at least 30 minutes of specific exercise. Basically, any kind of exercise helps to activate the lymphatic system. Besides swimming and running, you can swing and bounce on a mini-trampoline as a very effective way to cleanse the lymphatic system. It also has the advantage of activating deeper-lying lymphatic vessels. A recommended routine is to exercise for ten minutes three times a day. Since a trampoline is normally placed within your own four walls, it can be used at any time without much ado.

Skipping is another good way to keep the lymph circulating, but even slow, flowing movements together with deep conscious breathing activate and stimulate the flow of lymph, so for instance yoga, qi gong and tai chi can be used for this purpose.

The spine too should be kept flexible, to stimulate the flow of cerebrospinal fluid in the spinal cord. This can be done by using rippling or spiral movements, both of which are basic parts of yoga. They not only stimulate the fluid in the spine but also keep the spine flexible, strong and energetic.

Basically, the exercise should be gentle and moderate rather than strenuous and exhausting, which is neither useful nor necessary. Sports with abrupt movements like tennis or squash are less helpful, but otherwise moving a lot in the fresh air stimulates the natural drainage of lymph. The lymphatic system benefits from every kind of natural movement, as it is thereby massaged and kept healthy. A list of relevant sports is provided in the chapter *Regular Lymphatic Activation.*

Mini-trampoline

A mini-trampoline is a simple and effective accessory for keeping the lymph moving. Without any strain or needless sweating, you can resort to it for stimulating the lymphatic system. You need only swing and bounce for the system to be effectively cleansed. There is no need to jump high, as jumping up and down a little is enough. This is because the continual change from less weight to more weight on the vascular system ensures a constant change of relaxation and tension of the musculature and also activates the deeper-lying lymphatic vessels.

Exercise on the mini-trampoline is thus like a lymphatic drainage for the whole body, and at the same time the jumping up and down strengthens the muscles. A strong musculature furthers the flow of lymph, so training on the trampoline benefits the system both ways.

It is a good idea to train for tent to twenty minutes a day, which should be possible with a trampoline at home. If you find it hard to balance while bouncing, you can place the trampoline near something to hold onto, or you can buy a trampoline with things to hold onto already. Anyone who, for health reasons, feels unable to bounce on a mini-trampoline can use one for walking, as this too helps to get the lymph flowing.

After training on the trampoline, you should remember to drink enough. Bouncing on a trampoline is not especially tiring, so the need for more drink is easily forgotten, not only to replace the water lost but also to activate and detoxify the lymphatic system.

Skipping

The most popular game among children may be skipping, which after all is only child's play and easily done. But what is easy for children is also good for grown-ups in improving the lymphatic system. It also improves the cardiovascular system and is an excellent way to lose weight. The improvement of the lymphatic system is due to the fact that jumping and the associated body tension compress the body, but skipping does even more. As a holistic workout, it positively affects your condition, coordination, sense of balance and the muscles of your pelvic floor and legs.

Another advantage of skipping is that it can be done at any time at home, so you are not constrained by the weather or by times available in a gym. All you need is a rope and gym shoes, or you can even skip barefoot. The length of rope needed depends on your height. At first, the rope may tangle or you may not hop high enough, but beginnings are mostly the trickiest part.

Detox yoga

Apart from being generally good for the health, some yoga exercises also further the detoxification of the lymph in particular. Rotary movements and bending forward purify the body by acting like an inner massage. These cleansing exercises stimulate lymphatic activity, letting the system cope more with detoxification. For instance there is the pose called the lord of the fishes, in which the pelvis and legs are twisted to one side, and the pose called the forceps, in which you sit on the ground with your legs stretched out and try to touch your toes.

These exercises also improve the metabolism, the blood circulation and the digestion, ridding the body of pollutants and waste products. Even so called yogic flows, in which one movement leads to another, help the blood to circulate and the body to be detoxified, an example being the greeting to the sun (surya namaskar).

Two other suitable exercises are the ones called the crocodile and the frog. They massage and stimulate the detoxification organs and clear the mind of negative thoughts, effectively detoxifying the mind too. In fact, they further the self-healing powers of the body as a whole. Likewise all exercises placing the body upside down, like the head-stand (sirsasana) and shoulder-stand (saravangasana) stimulate the lymphatic system. This is because the lymph flows backwards during the exercises then flows forwards again into the lymph nodes, where it is cleansed and detoxified.

You can also support the lymphatic system by twisting in the half fish pose (ardha matsyendrasana) and the revolved chair pose (parivtta utkatasana). Toxins and pathogens are wrung out of the body like dirt out of a floor-cloth. Twisting the spine, as in performing the 'eight movements of the spine', likewise provides basic detoxification and strengthen the body, and Kapalabhati breathing, a kind of yogic snorting, is likewise very effective.

Special gymnastics

There are many simple gymnastics exercises for activating the lymph:

Stand in front of a chair you can hold onto. Rise slowly onto your tiptoes then sink back onto the soles of your feet. Repeat 15 times.

You may also do this exercise while lying on your back and lifting your legs as high as you can without strain. Curl the toes up on one foot slowly then slowly relax them again, then do the same with the other foot. Repeat 8 times with each foot.

You may prefer to sit on a chair and do the exercise slowly 15 times altogether.

You may sit upright on a chair with your legs parted as wide as your hips then let both feet rest on their heels then on their toes.

Controlled breathing

Deliberately deep breathing as well as the fire breath purifies and cleanses the lymphatic system. The lymph flows again or more than it did. Proper breathing is essential for stimulating the lymph, as it can increase the efficiency of cleansing more than tenfold.

Deep breathing activates the rib-cage and diaphragm, creating differences in pressure, which in turn cause the lymph to flow better. Deep breathing also cleanses other organs of detoxification and improves their efficiency by supplying them with oxygen and energy.

Swift, shallow breathing on the other hand supplies the body with less oxygen and relieves it of less carbon dioxide, so the blood becomes more acidic and hinders detoxification. Generally, we breathe too swiftly and shallowly, especially when under stress.

The boons of breathing well

We all breathe, but few of us think about it and do so properly, though proper breathing is a wonderful and often neglected source of health and well being. Breathing is an enormous source of energy. A restful and even flow of breath into and out of the belly relieves nervousness, restlessness, anxiety and tension in a very short time. We only have to remind ourselves how to breathe properly by using not only the chest but also the belly for the sake of enough oxygen.

Poor breathing is often due to a poor quality of life. If you sit dejectedly in front of a computer, unable to solve this or that problem, your breathing automatically becomes swift and shallow. Your belly may also tense up, hindering the diaphragm. Indeed, in front of a computer, we often forget about how we are sitting, so our backs hunch and our necks tense up.

Mental problems like fear, depression and the stress of deadlines and multi-tasking make proper breathing as hard as running the gauntlet. This has given rise to expressions like '**It takes my breath away**' or '**It's enough to choke you**'. These expressions underline how closely connected the mind and body are. Mental stress can affect the breathing, then the breathing can affect the mind, so things go from bad to worse.

Let us take anxiety for instance. If we experience a shock, our breathing stops of its own accord, and this only increases the fear. Stress can literally take out breath away, but normally we tend to pay it little attention. Many people treat breathing as a natural instinct in need of no special tuition, so they overlook its importance till feeling the effects of poor breathing.

This can lead to a whole set of ailments like depression, insomnia, headaches, and problems with the circulation or digestion, so it is important to learn to breathe slowly, calmly and rhythmically. Hence therapists tend to say: '**We shall let the breath come and go**.' Breathing should not only happen but also be experienced and cherished.

Breathing properly does wonders for your vitality, harmonizes body and soul and brings them to equilibrium. It improves your powers of self-healing and the supply of oxygen to your body. You begin to feel livelier and fit, and your body is able to relax deeply. Quiet, continual breathing into the belly can help the lungs to work better and can eliminate more pollutants.

It is useful to learn without stress how to breathe well. You can then practice it covertly in everyday situations. Especially if we are under stress, our breaths become fast and shallow, but these are the very times when we should try to breathe deeply and slowly, to supply the body with enough oxygen and to lessen our inner tension. When we are breathing deeply deliberately, the belly swells as air come in and sinks as air goes out, as does the abdominal wall.

It is important to breathe calmly, deeply and slowly, then during the exercise you will notice that your mind and body become calmer and relaxed too. It is best to practice once a day 10 times for about 2 minutes a time. Sit or lie down and ensure that everything around you is restful. Shut your eyes then breathe slowly through your nose and let the air flow into your belly. While breathing in, count to at least five or preferably up to ten, then breathe out slowly. Let your breath flow freely without being noticeably squeezed in or out and repeat the exercise 10 to 15 times.

The meaning of breathing

Breathing is an innate reflex which hardly anyone has questioned. Nonetheless, the importance of breathing often comes to attention as shown by expressions like '**It takes my breath away**' or '**The fear is enough to choke me**', if something is startling or dreadful. Someone who sighs deeply may have to be patient, and '**I feel stifled**' may not always be a request for the windows to be opened. It may rather express the effect of one person on another. '**I need to take a breather**' is mostly a sign that someone is overworked. But feeling breathless may not always have a negative connotation, as a couple freshly in love may likewise feel their breath taken away by each other's presence.

How we live, eat, act, sleep and sit tallies with how we breathe. As a rule, it is only when things go wrong with us physically or mentally, especially with the channels for the breath, that we consciously think about breathing. Even then, the treatment often consists only in taking medicine, but there is no need to reinvent the wheel, since mankind has known about the healing power of the breath for thousands of years. In India the yogis teach how best to breathe while meditating, and in China

qigong is used to strengthen the universal life-force through breathing. Indeed nearly all religions are familiar with the spiritual healing power of energetic breathing.

Breathing & healing

To most scientists, breathing is only a mechanical process stimulated by the so-called partial pressure. This is the pressure gradient between carbon dioxide and oxygen. But breathing is much more than merely acquiring oxygen and releasing carbon dioxide, as shown by the fact that we can live for about 40 days without food and 5 days without water but only a few minutes without air.

About 21% of the air is made up of oxygen, which the body needs to burn nutrients. Only in this way can the organisms and its numerous functions be maintained. The brain is very sensitive to a lack of oxygen, and if supplied with too little, it immediately works less well and some brain cells die within three minutes. From catching a cold, most of us know how unpleasant it is not to be able to breathe well.

The lungs are the organs where gases are exchanged between the body and the surrounding air. Air flows into the lungs though the mouth and throat and from there into the trachea and bronchi. The bronchi divide and subdivide into continually thinner branches called the bronchioles, and from them air passes into air sacs known as alveoli.

These sacs can be pictured as very small protuberances crossed by very thin walls. Everyone has about 300 million of them, so if they were spread out and placed next to each other, the area covered would be about the size of a soccer field. Only in the alveoli does the air exchange gases with the blood, which takes oxygen in and bears it through the whole body. As a waste product, carbon dioxide is released into the alveoli and breathed out.

The alveoli are very sensitive and fare best on clean, slightly humid air at a comfortable temperature. This is why the widely branched bronchial system is lined with mucous membranes, which also protect the bronchi from invading pathogens. On these membranes, there are goblet cells, which secrete tough mucous, forming a film on the surface. But most of the cells there have fine hairs or cilia on them. The cilia move to and fro, taking dust, bacteria and viruses away from the breathing system, as if along an assembly line. Consequently, a certain amount of mucous gets into the throat but is soon swallowed by reflex. Germs in the mucous thus pass into the stomach, where they are rendered harmless by gastric acid.

A grown up normally breathes in and out about 12 to 18 times a minute, and children two or three times as often. Every breath amounts to about half a liter of air, so 6 to 9 liters are breathed in and out per minute or about 10 000 liters a day. Between the ages of 20 and 30, the average lung volume is 4 liters, and by the age of 60 it has become just under 2. In the course of a lifetime, the average consumption of oxygen is 20 000 000 liters. Basically, breathing is the most natural thing in the world, so breathing is one of the bodily processes taken for granted, as long they work well.

Unfortunately, in the modern world, most people have forgotten how to breathe naturally, using both the chest and the belly. Faulty breathing impairs the motory system, the cardiovascular system and the lung system. There are many reasons for breathing poorly, one of the main ones being a poor posture. In sitting at a desk for a long time, we tend to slump over the desk. We then breathe too shallowly, not into the belly, but at other times – when looking at the television for instance – we can try to improve.

Few people are even aware that they breath poorly, though there are warning signs, especially tension in the chest and back. We then feel restricted in our movements and even that we are unable to breathe thoroughly and are often short of breath. Even the rhythm of breathing may be affected, as the shallower the breathing, the faster it becomes. It may sound like a wheeze or whistle and even stop, and poor breathing may even cause a persistent cough.

Shallow breathing not only leads to a feeling of tightness and tension, it also lessens the amount of oxygen supplied to the body, as less reaches the blood vessels in the lower part of the lungs. If breathing is less than ideal, it often leads to chronic fatigue and poorer performance, so correct breathing has to be relearned and is then a wonderful source of health and well-being. The key to sustainable health is breathing deeply into the belly. As much air as possible is then drawn into the lungs, supplying every cell in the body with oxygen, and the effect is immediately soothing.

If we breathe more deeply into our bellies, we can focus more on our work and have more vitality, endurance and ability to perform tasks. This is why correct breathing is indispensable for brain-workers as well as for top athletes. In other words, our unused potential for our lives and aims can be realized once poor breathing has been corrected. Indeed, many complaints and ailments can be cured or alleviated if breathing improves and becomes more functional.

To keep in mind how strongly outer circumstances can influence the healthy rhythm of breathing, it is useful to note the two metaphors *'fear keeps air away'* and *'stress strangles the throat'*. Without fear and stress, oxygen-enriched blood can reach all cells in the body extremely fast, then toxins and slags are led out of the body. If breathing is shallow and gives the blood too little oxygen, the blood corpuscles stick together and may hinder the flow of lymph. Toxins are then inadequately flushed out and nutrients and other vital materials fail to reach their destinations.

This may even cause toxins to be dumped in various 'depots' and in the joints, where they may cause inflammation and other complaints. The body cells also have to do more to compensate for the lack of oxygen due to poor breathing. If too little oxygen is circulating in the blood to meet cells' needs, more poisons are stored in the cell fluid. This may cause the whole body to swell, and especially stressed parts may become inflamed.

Training the muscles used in breathing is also the best protection against infections. If the respiratory tract – the most important portal of entry for pathogens of all kinds – is well aired, viruses and bacteria find it hard to stick to it and multiply.

If we catch our breath in the proverbial sense, it is time to remove the blockages and to restore the natural flow. This improves physical and mental health and releases valuable resources of energy. In freeing your breath, you also free yourself in many respects, as it not only calms your body but also endows it with more power. Your perceptions become more open and clearer, and the grounding is often followed by an inner awakening.

In conventional medicine, this transcendental component of breathing is not taken into account, so a lot of healing potential remains unrealized. The energetic-spiritual aspect of proper breathing is no esoteric hocus-pocus of recent vintage. Already in the Vedas from thousands of years ago, the right breathing for the unity of body, mind and soul is described. There are now new psycho-therapeutic and alternative medical approaches in the theory of breathing, but even old knowledge is increasingly coming to light, such as the influence of the sun and moon on breathing.

Fire-breathing

Fire-breathing is a special form of cleansing and is able to detoxify the body thoroughly. This kind of breathing is very fast, so the lungs are cleansed and the oxygen content of the blood is greatly increased.

The capacity of the lungs increases and the circulation and cardiac activity improve.

The airways are thoroughly cleansed, so fire-breathing is good for treating hay fever, asthma, congested or inflamed sinuses and colds. Moreover, the liver, heart and stomach are usefully massaged. The whole body is cleansed and purified and metabolic processes are improved. The solar plexus is activated and the inner fire is stimulated.

Usually, the fast breathing is done while sitting, but it can also be done while standing or walking. There is a clear emphasis on breathing out, which is powerful and active, while breathing in is passive and reflexive. Attention is paid only to breathing out, and breathing in is automatic.

It is the forceful breathing out which is powerfully purifying. The wall of the belly rises while breathing in and falls while breathing out, but the breathing remains deep and relaxed. You start with about 20 breaths and go on in the course of time to take 40 to 60. During the exercise, the head and upper body are to remain at rest and only the wall of the belly is to move. Fire-breathing is often combined with alternative breathing, which is practiced afterwards.

Fast breathing is also used to alter the state of consciousness. Your head feels empty and free and your thoughts fade, so rapid breathing can also be used as a prelude to meditation.

Lymphatic massages

A lymphatic massage is a massage in which the skin is stimulated for the sake of the tissue fluid. Unlike many common forms of massage, lymphatic massage is gentle and harmonious. The skin is neither firmly kneaded nor intensively worked on. Lymphatic massage is used to detoxify and purify the body and to activate the lymphatic system. It is a gentle form of lymphatic drainage and stimulates the lymphatic system but is usually applied to only certain parts of the body.

Both lymphatic massage and lymphatic drainage should be performed by specially trained physiotherapists. An effective lymph massage lasts at least 30 minutes, as it takes time for the sluggish lymph to flow faster. Massaging is always done without cream, and in the case of very dry skin, it may be useful to use a top quality oil. The massage should take place in a calm and pleasant atmosphere. As a rule, the neck is the first part of the body to be massaged, which has to do with the direction the lymph flows in.

During the lymphatic massage, the lymphatic channels and lymph nodes are massaged, whereby various grips are applied. A certain technique, which exerts pressure on the lymph nodes and the lymphatics can strengthen the cleansing function of the lymphatic system. The pressure is constantly changed, and the various grips are applied slowly and rhythmically. The skin is gently stretched to let the fluid be channeled from the tissue into the lymphatic vessels.

The massage is continued with movements in the form of waves and circles as well as with pumping and twisting movements. This activates and detoxifies the lymphatic system, further pushing the lymph in its natural direction of flow, which increased the lymphatic drainage many times over. As a part of a detoxification cure, lymphatic massages can be performed two or three times a week or even once a day.

A special kind of lymphatic massage is the Ayurvedic herbal stamp massage Jambira Pinda Sweda, which is used to purify and detoxify the body and to stimulate the organism. The circular and stroking movements stimulate the flow of lymph and also the metabolism, then after the massage a client should drink enough.

Lymphatic drainage is performed if edema is present in certain parts of the body such as the arms and legs. For instance, after breast surgery, quite a few women suffer from edema in their arms, due to the removal of lymph nodes in their armpits. Lymphatic drainage, preferably once a day, and compression therapy together let the swelling of the arms subside again and also ease the pain.

People with lipolymph edema likewise benefit from lymphatic drainage. In this mostly congenital ailment there are fat deposits in the legs, hindering the flow of lymph. Lymph drainage can also be usefully applied to sports injuries and venous insufficiency. In the case of a stubborn cold, the lymph nodes on the neck can be massaged. The swelling on the neck then subsides, the complaints are relieved and the healing is faster.

Lymphatic drainage should not be used for thrombosis, severe cardiac insufficiency, thyroid disease, malignant tumors still to be operated on, asthma, acute infections and acute eczema, nor should it be used during pregnancy. Lymphatic massages should not be performed at home without prior instruction, as it may otherwise be performed too intensively.

Detox turbo cupping

In the traditional procedure cupping glasses are used, which are heated internally then applied. As the cups cool, the air in them applies less pressure to the skin, effectively sucking. The classical procedure activates certain reflex zones on the back, which in turn affect the tallying inner organs and systems of organs.

The therapist begins by feeling the patient's back, to make out any bumps or hollows implying that the tallying organs are malfunctioning, then a glass is placed on the skin and effectively sucks at it. This is also known as dry cupping. The powerful suction increases the flow of blood, removing slag, toxins and other debris from the body.

The local drainage of the blood eliminates whatever may be hindering the flow of blood so has a strong detoxification effect. The circulation of the blood and lymph is stimulated, as are all organs, including the immune system. Through the action of the stimulus on the body, fluid dammed in tissues is released, as are further tensions and blockages. The whole flow of energy through the body is reactivated and all cells are supplied with fresh energy. Cupping may be used not only for detoxification but also for back pain, tension, rheumatic complaints, indigestion, chronic fatigue and weakness.

In bloody cupping, the skin is cut with a small knife then the cups are applied to the skin. The idea is to let any blood present in the congested tissues escape together with the pollutants. This also thins the blood, so lets it become more fluid. If the blood has already been thinned, due to surgery or disorders of the blood, this method should not be used. Dry cupping is generally used for chronic discomfort or prevention, and bloody cupping for acute problems already painful. If bloody cupping is used, attention should be paid to hygiene, so as not to infect the cuts.

Acupuncture massage

The so-called acupuncture massage according to Penzel is performed without needles and is suitable for letting the lymph flow again. During this massage, the meridians (energy channels) and the acupuncture points are treated with a metal stick. This frees the body's energy system from blockages and disturbances, letting the energy flow freely again. It also stimulates the circulation of the lymph, intensifying the detoxification.

Dry brush massage

A classical way to counter toxins and a hardening of the body is the dry brush massage, which also improves general well being. Regular massages with a brush stimulate the whole metabolism, strengthen the body's resiliance, increase the circulation of the blood, invigorate the organism and improve the skin structure. On the one hand a brush massage directly affects the skin and on the other hand it also affects the nerve tracts and thus the release of substances used for signaling. By stabilizing the autonomous nervous system, the massage also calms and harmonizes the heartbeat and blood pressure. The mind calms down as well, and inner tension and nervousness subside.

Through the intensive contact and movement of deeper skin and muscle layers, the circulation of the blood is stimulated, so the whole organism is revitalized and regains its zest. This increases the supply of fresh blood together with oxygen, nutrients and antibodies to all organs. It stimulates not only the metabolism but also the lymphatic system, so harmful substances are washed away and eliminated faster.

Dry brushing also optimally affects lymphatic capillaries just below the skin and helps the lymph to flow. The activity of the lymph nodes is likewise stimulated, letting them better fulfill their function of detoxification. Pores of the skin open when brushed, letting poisons and slag be eliminated through the skin, so dry brushing also supports this route of detoxification.

The massage should always begin with the extremities of the body and move towards the heart, as this improves the flow of blood back to it. All materials no longer needed or even harmful are thereby removed from the massaged tissue, improving or regenerating cells and organs. It should not be applied to skin affected by inflammatory, allergic or infectious ailments or in the case of degenerative vascular ailments (like varicose veins), neurasthenia and thyroid disorders, and if applied in the evening, it may later disturb sleep.

A brush massage lasting about ten to twenty minutes daily or every two or three days is optimal for health. A massage should ideally be applied in the morning, arousing the sluggish organism and stimulating the activity of the lymphatic system. The brush should have firm and clean natural bristles, for instance from plant fiber. Strong brushing is neither helpful nor needed, so if the brushing is felt to be unpleasant, it should be changed.

A long-handled brush is useful to reach less accessible parts of the body like the back. The brush should be kept dry so not be used while bathing or showering, but after being brushed, you should take a warm bath if possible for about twenty minutes. This too is a help in detoxifying the body. You may instead take a cold shower after the brush massage.

Instructions

The brush massage should always be towards the heart. Heavy rubbing should be avoided and replaced by long strokes or, in the case of some parts of the body, by circular movements.

At first, circular movements are applied to the feet, beginning with the outside of the right foot.
The same is then done to the instep.
The procedure is repeated, beginning with the outside of the left foot.
Circular movements are applied to the front and back, inner and outer sides of the calves and thighs.
The legs are then brushed ten times from the ankles upwards.
Circular movements are also applied to the buttocks.
Brush strokes are applied to the back of the right hand and continue along the arm to the shoulder. The inside of the arm is likewise massaged from the hand upwards.
The same is then done to the left hand and arm.
Each armpit is thereby massaged ten times with circular movements.
Circular movements are also applied to the belly and chest, massaging the belly is massaged according to the course of the colon from the bottom right to the bottom left.
Movements in the form of the figure 8 are applied to the chest.
Finally the brush is stroked downwards along the nape, though not specifically towards the heart.
The face may be brushed additionally, but this calls for a special brush.

Contrast therapy

Dousing yourself with hot and cold water in alternation stimulates the whole circulatory system, improves blood circulation in the organs and has a positive effect on the immune system. It is good for the health, especially in detoxifying the whole body. It also improves breathing, letting it become deeper and better and letting cramped bronchial muscles relax. It also calms an over-excited nervous system. All in all, contrast bath or shower therapy is good for the whole body and leaves you feeling as if you were newly born.

Start a contrast shower with very hot water for up to two minutes then switch to very cold water for up to one minute. Repeat this procedure a few times then round it off with cold water. If you are new to this procedure, it is best to get used to it slowly. Avoid extreme temperatures and staying in one phase for too long. Instead, switch phases at shorter intervals, to give your body enough time to get used to the procedure.

If the extreme temperatures are too much for you at first, just point the nozzle of the shower towards your feet and arms, then slowly extend the area of application to include the legs and back. Include your belly last, as it is more sensitive.

Contrast baths or showers supply the body with fresh blood and oxygen and also remove accumulations of toxins and pathogens from parts not otherwise reached by enough blood. The alternation of cold and warm water hardens, irrigates and detoxifies the body and strengthens the immune system. The temperature stimuli are mediated through the skin and trigger positive reactions. Blood vessels contract in reaction to the cold phase and dilate in reaction to the warm one, stimulating the circulation of the blood through all the body. This activates the metabolism, letting all kinds of harmful materials be washed away.

The changes of temperature also activate the lymphatic vessels, letting lymph be taken away faster. Blockages in the lymphatic system are removed, so the lymph can flow freely. The narrowing and widening of the vessels presses all kinds of pollutants out of the body, so a contrast bath or shower has a wonderfully regenerating and cleansing effect on the system. It also improves the blood pressure, as blood vessels are likewise narrowed and widened, helping them to stay elastic.

The temperature in the cold phase should lie between 10° and 16°C and in the warm phase between 36° and 39°C, but extreme cold should be avoided if you happen to have high blood pressure, or it will become even higher. The same applies to people who are elderly or otherwise frail, due for instance to heart failure. If your blood pressure is very high, you should avoid this kind of therapy altogether to be on the safe side.

Treading water

If you tread water while wading through cold water, you strengthen your immune system, activate your metabolism and improve your circulation. Treading water is both refreshing and relaxing, so the autonomous nervous system is calmed and the blood pressure lowered. In particular, treading water lessens blockages in the lymphatic system, improving the flow of lymph and the return of blood to the heart through the venous system.

For treading, fill the bath to a hand's breadth below the hollow of the knee with cold water then walk through the water like a stork. When your weight is on one leg, lift the other one wholly out of the water and let the foot point down. If the cold becomes too much, end the procedure. For all cold water applications, the body must be warm. At need, you must warm it up beforehand by doing gymnastics for instance. It is no less important to warm the body again afterwards. Warm socks and a cozy lie in bed may be enough. The treatment is soothing and relaxing so is a good preparation for going to bed in the evening for a healthy sleep.

In many spas there are Kneipp pools where you can alternate between walking through warm water at 35°C and cool water at 15°C. There are also Kneipp pools in many parks for treading water in the open air. But you can also try wherever water is flowing through the countryside. Treading water is unsuitable for people menstruating or with kidney, bladder or other abdominal complaints.

Cold hosing the body

For activating or detoxifying the lymphatic system, you can also hose water over yourself like over your arms and thighs. The effect is effervescent and invigorating. Cold hosing is especially valued for improving and strengthening the lymphatic system.

What do you need to do it?

A rubber hose attached to a shower or tap.

What should you heed in doing it?

The temperature of the water should ideally be 18°C.
If this is too cool for you, try a moderate temperature of 18°C to 22°C.
It should not be done in a cold or drafty room.
The hose should be held to let water pour gently over your skin without bouncing off it.
The hose should be held about 5 to 10 cm from the skin.
After being hosed, the arms or legs are not dried. The water is only brushed off, then the moist skin is covered with a cloth of natural fibers.

Cold hosing should not be done just after a meal or physical exercise.

Cold hosing should be done no longer than is felt to be pleasant.

The body should then be warmed up again, for instance by lying in bed or by doing gymnastics.

Cold hosing the thighs

This stimulates the body, especially the blood circulation and the metabolism and has a purifying effect. In particular the lymphatic system is stimulated, relieved and detoxified. The nervous system too is calmed, which is why cold hosing the thighs may make you sleepy. Cold hosing the thighs can also be used to reduce varicose veins, water retention in the legs and bruising. It also eases headaches, high blood pressure and constipation. It should not be used for infections of the urinary tract, chills, heart disease or open wounds in the areas treated, sciatic nerve pain or menstruation.

How to do it

Begin with the right foot then move slowly up the outside of the leg to the hipbone. Then hose the inside of the leg from the groin down. The same is then to be done to the left leg.

Cold hosing the arms

This is refreshing and stimulates the circulation so is especially helpful in reducing weariness, exhaustion and hypotension. It also detoxifies the lymphatic system and offers relief but should not be used in the case of cardiac arrhythmia or bronchial asthma.

How to do it

Begin with the back of the right hand then guide the jet of water along the outside of the arm to the shoulder and back along the inside of the arm to the palm of the hand then do the same with the left hand and arm. It is a good idea to do some gymnastics afterwards to warm the arms up again.

Alkaline baths

These detoxify the body through the skin. They help the lymph to flow, to achieve a balanced state and to rid itself of poisons.

How to take one

A small but not too small amount of alkaline salt should be added to the bathwater. This should then reach a pH value between 8.5 and 9.5, to be checked with litmus paper. Often we are advised to take only a few tablespoonfuls of the salts, but this may be too little. Owing to osmosis, acids in the body are neutralized by the added alkali and thereby eliminated. The principle behind it is that if the pH values on each side of a permeable membrane differ greatly, osmosis lessens the difference.

In effect the alkali in the bath draws the acids out of the body through the skin. The temperature of the bath should lie between 35°C and 38°C and higher temperatures should be avoided, so as not to stress the circulation and the heart. For the osmotic effect to be enough, it is useful to bathe for about an hour followed by about two hours of rest. After bathing, you should not take a shower but let the skin dry naturally or dab it gently with a cloth, to let the alkali continue to affect it.

Saunas

A sauna is very effective in detoxifying the body, as sweating not only stimulates the metabolism but also detoxifies it. Naturopaths claim that you can become healthy only by sweating enough. Visits to a sauna cleanse and activate the lymphatic system and are always a welcome option if no ailments pose a risk. Owing to the increased flow of blood and the alternating cold and hot temperatures, the lymphatic vessels are caused to contract and dilate, increasing the flow of lymph and improving detoxification in the lymph nodes.

Sweating causes pores in the skin to open, letting harmful materials and toxins be released. This too accords with a basic principle of naturopathy, according to which waste should firstly be removed from the so-called noble organs like the heart and liver and be passed on to the so-called base organs like the skin and mucous membranes. In view of all these benefits, saunas should not be visited only in winter. A sauna is a treat for the body and soul in all seasons, enabling them to relax and rest, even in times of stress.

The immune system too benefits from regular visits to the sauna, as the varying temperatures train and harden the body, forming a bulwark against colds and influenza. Regular visits to the sauna also improve its ability to cope with fluctuations of temperature. Alternating cold and warm stimuli invigorate and detoxify it, leaving it tough and resilient. Exposure to dry air of up to 100°C increases the circulation of the blood, and there is a swift increase in the number of cells removing end products of the metabolism, toxins, slags and bacteria.

After a sauna session, there is a need for enough cooling, or the effect of the sauna is less. Cooling the body stabilizes the circulation, draws fresh and unused air into the lungs, and increases the oxygen content of the blood. The sweat baths should be short and intense, amounting to about 8-12 minutes), then you should step out into the fresh air. It is a good idea to pour cold water over yourself, to plunge into a pool or to have a foot bath. You should take a break of at least 15 minutes between the separate sauna sessions and treat yourself to at least half an hour's rest at the end. After a session, remember to drink enough water or fruit-juice with mineral water.

In general, and especially as a beginner, you should take care not to overdo it. Pay attention to your body, as saunas do not have to be long to be effective. Moreover, you should not go to a sauna if you have been rushing around, have a full stomach or are tipsy. You should also not go to a sauna if your blood pressure is unstable or if you have cardiac arrhythmia, diseases of the heart, thyroid hyperfunction, acute or chronic infections, gastric or intestinal ulcers, epilepsy or multiple sclerosis. If in doubt, ask a doctor.

Loose clothing

Avoid tight clothing for the sake of your lymph. If clothing is too tight, the lymph channels are squeezed and the lymph can no longer flow freely without disturbance. It is better to wear pleasantly loose clothing which lets the skin breathe. Women should wear bras with comfortable straps which do not curl and are wide enough not to cut into the skin. The band under the breasts should be soft, wide and not restrictive, and no bra should be worn during the night.

Briefs with a tight waistband should not be worn at all, and elastic bands on pants and skirts should not be fastened or exert pressure. Neither belts on dresses nor seat-belts in cars should dig into you. If possible, wear flat shoes without high heels, because heels more than four centimeters high hinder the flow of blood back to the heart. You should avoid footwear like rubber boots, which stop air reaching the feet.

Compression stockings

These encourage the flow of lymph by creating a pressure gradient from the ankles to the top of the legs. This prevents the lymph from flowing backwards or stagnating in the tissues. Ideally the stockings should be made to measure, to fit perfectly. They should be worn regularly during the day and can be taken off at night. Dressing aids may make it easier to pull the stockings on.

Compression products range from knee stockings to thigh stockings and tights. They are available in four classes, defined in terms of the pressure exerted round the ankles. Compression dressings made up of short-stretch bandages have the advantage of being separately adjustable, but applying them is rather tricky, so they should rather be applied by specially trained therapists.

Risky deodorants

Deodorants hinder detoxification of the lymph, especially if they contain aluminum compounds to seal the sweat ducts. In the long term, this can make the body acidic and let the ducts be blocked by other pollutants too. Our main lymph nodes are in the armpits, so blocking the sweat ducts there may not only overload the body with pollutants but also cause serious ailments. There is even some evidence that the use of deodorants containing aluminum may cause breast cancer.

What should we do about it? We hardly wish to leave a personal stench in the air behind us or to see crowds thinning away at our approach, but we are not doomed to do so. This can mainly be avoided by regularly shaving the hair under our arms, since the overall surface area of the hair is huge and accommodating to bacteria. Their waste products are the source of smells, so removing the hair and the bacteria with them tackles the roots of the problem.

It is also better to use a deodorant than to use an antiperspirant. A deodorant merely neutralizes smells, whereas an antiperspirant locks toxins up in the body. It is also useful to wear cotton clothing, which air is able to seep through, than to wear tight synthetic clothing. The latter only makes you sweat excessively and soon becomes smelly.

Further tips

Avoid crossing your legs, as this hinders the flow of blood.
Avoid the two Ss (standing and sitting) and favor the two Rs (reclining and running).
Lift your legs as often as possible.
At night let your legs be slightly higher than your body, to let blood flow back to your heart.
Let your feet and legs change their positions as often as they wish, and let your feet circle or rock.
Begin each day by lifting your legs while still in bed.

'Cycling'

Flex your feet now and then, even under an office table or on an aircraft.
Carry no heavy loads.
Try to limit your weight.
Remember: the less you smoke, the better.
Avoid stress.
Favor vegetables and fruits over meat and sausages.

Excess acid & lymph congestion

Too much acid over a long period deregulates the lymphatic system. Acid-producing foods gradually weaken the system and cause it to work less well.

All of its functions, such as supplying cells with nutrients and detoxifying and maintaining the immune system, depend on the extent of acidity. If the system becomes and remains too acidic, the lymphatic vessels become porous and brittle, leading to lymphatic congestion and inflammatory reactions.

It is therefore a good idea to choose a diet with a bias towards alkalies by favoring plenty of vegetables and fruit and fresh unprocessed foods. Highly processed foods, fast foods and sweets overload our bodies with acids, slag and other pollutants. Meat should seldom be eaten and pork avoided. The opposite is true of celery juice, a glass of which you may drink before any meal, to detoxify and stimulate the lymphatic system.

Once the lymph has become too acidic, it cannot flow properly and may become congested. The shape of the lymphatic vessels changes and the flow of the lymph is blocked by slags and toxins, gradually poisoning the body. The signs may be acute or chronic in the form of ailments like digestive problems, headache, eczema, cellulite, edema, heavy legs, muscle pain, loss of performance, chronic bronchitis, colds and inflammation of the sinuses and tonsils.

In the long term there may be asthma, harm to the veins, arthrosis, arthritis, joint and connective tissue diseases, rheumatism or gout. There may also be higher blood pressure and more weight. The problem in diagnosis is that the first signs may not point unambiguously to the lymphatic system, as other causes have similar effects. It becomes clear that something has gone wrong with the body but not why. Malfunctioning of the lymphatic system also affects the immune system, so you may have continual infections.

An acidic environment also solidifies proteins in the lymph, blocking the flow of lymph and leading to further congestion. In other words an acidic environment blocks the flow of lymph, and the blocked flow makes the environment more acidic , so things go from bad to worse.

Acid-producing foods include meat and animal products, milk and dairy products (except butter), cereals, fats and oils, sugars, alcoholic drinks and so on. For more information about this, please read the chapter about the regulation of acids and alkalies below. The ratio of acids to alkalies may be improved by moderately exercising and by avoiding all stress, as explained in more detail in the chapters on how to lessen stress and to relax.

Too much fat and protein

To safeguard the lymphatic system, we should favor a low-protein and -fat diet. Big protein and fat molecules cannot always be borne by the bloodstream, so this thankless task has to be taken over by the lymphatic system. Protein has the property of drawing water to itself like iron filings to a magnet, then it absorbs the water like a sponge. The swollen and clumped protein molecules then litter the lymphatic vessels and hinder the flow of lymph.

The lymph becomes thicker and more solid, till cells are no longer supplied with enough nutrients, and toxins, slags, pathogens and old cells stay in the lymph too long or indefinitely due to the congestion, instead of being borne to the nodes, where they can be properly disposed of.

Sometimes the lymph stores the slags and toxins in the connective tissue as a last resort, to stop them poisoning the body straightaway, but this only passes the poisons on from one part of the body to another instead of solving the problem. The lymph is no longer clear and healthy but sticky, viscous, sluggish and slimy.

The effect of having too many saturated fats (lipids) in the diet is not much better. These too settle down in the lymph, where their big and unwieldy molecules stand in the way of its flow. This firstly hinders the flow and may later block it, causing it to stagnate. You should rather switch to a diet healthier for the lymph by choosing a diet biased towards alkalies with plenty of fruit, greens and salads.

Saturated fats and animal protein have an acidifying effect on the body so should be consumed only in moderation. The same applies to all kinds of sweets such as cake and chocolate. Salt should be used sparingly as it binds water in the body, causing fluid to pool in the tissues. Too much food is a burden on the lymphatic system and the body, so meals should not be too festive.

Regulating the lymphatic system

The basic medicine for helping the lymphatic system consists of drops or tablets (not to be taken if the thyroid gland is overactive). They are available from various producers of homeopathic medicine and are 'complex' remedies such as Lymphaden®, Lymphomyosot®, Lymphdiaral® and Jso Lymphmittel® in the sense of being blends of several homeopathic substances.

The effect can be enhanced by using a lymphatic ointment twice a day. Gently applying the ointment benefits the whole lymphatic system. You should apply it behind or under your ears and rub it with circular movements down towards your neck/lymph nodes and collarbone. Moreover, calcium carbonate is the key regulator of the lymphatic system and stimulates the flow of lymph.

Herbs for the lymph

Sweet clover

Yellow sweet clover (Latin: *Melilotus officinalis*) belongs to the family of butterfly plants (Latin: *Fabaceae*). This undemanding biennial herb is widespread in Europe and Asia and grows up to one meter in height. It can be found in fields and on the roadside, on railway tracks and in quarries as well as on scree and fallow land. In German it is known as Steinklee (stone clover) for being fond of stony places, and its Latin name may be due to the sweet honey-like scent of its flowers.

Meliloti herba is traditionally used in the form of tea or capsules, to stimulate the lymphatic system and to lessen lymphatic stress. In particular the coumarines in this clover release accumulated fluid and congestion in tissues. Moreover, it increases the circulation and the rate of flow in the venous and lymphatic systems and the resilience of blood vessels. It also makes capillaries less permeable and has an anti-inflammatory effect so can be used to treat not only chronic insufficiency and inflammation of the veins but also congestion or sluggishness of the lymph.

Tea can be made from it by pouring about 200 ml of water over a teaspoonful of the herb. After 10 minutes the herb is strained. The coumarines in the clover thin the blood, so the tea should not be taken with medicine inhibiting coagulation. For this reason, you should avoid too great a dose, but the dosage is hard to assess, as contents vary from plant to plant, so it is safer to take capsules.

Compresses

Compresses with yellow sweet clover can be applied externally. Compresses with *Meliloti herba* increase the circulation and the removal of lymph fluid from congested tissue. To prepare a compress, pour a liter of water over two tablespoonsful of yellow sweet clover and boil it for about 20 minutes. After straining, soak a bandage or compress with the extract, place it on the relevant part of the body and fasten it with another gauze bandage.

Sweet clover oil

This is good for the circulation and lessens congestion and edema. To produce the oil, the sweet clover is carefully minced then a high-quality vegetable oil (like olive or wheat-germ oil) is added to about 20 g of the crushed clover. The mixture is allowed to stand for four to six weeks but has to be shaken daily, to ensure that the active ingredients of the sweet clover pass into the oil. After straining, the oil is stored in a dark bottle. It is applied externally, then it stimulates the flow of lymph, helps weary legs and improves edema and ailments of the veins.

Cranesbill

To detoxify the lymph, you may use the best known member of the big group of cranesbills, *Geranium robertianum*. This is known variously in English as herb-Robin, red robin, death come quickly, storksbill, fox geranium, stinking Bob, squinter-pip, crow's foot or, in North America, Robert's geranium. The allusion to the bill of a crane or stork is due to the pointed shape of the fruit awns.

The varieties of cranesbill belong to the family of geraniums. There are altogether about 400 species found on all continents, including the Antarctic. They prefer a cool temperate climate and are able to thrive on moist soil. Most of these herbaceous species are perennial but some are annual or biennial. Robert's geranium is an annual plant with a height of 20-50 cm and can be used internally or externally in the form of compresses and ointments.

The ingredients of Robert's geranium include the bitter substance geraniin, tannins, flavanoids and essential oil. This herb has a purifying, detoxifying, astringent and dissolving effect. Physical and mental poisons are dissolved and drawn out of the body. In particular, Robert's geranium activates and stimulates the flow of lymph, detoxifying and purifying the lymphatic system.

Moreover, the herb can be used to strengthen the nerves, especially in states of anxiety or trauma, as the herb has a detoxifying effect on even the emotional plane. Shocks and mental toxins are dissolved and extracted. Owing to its astringent and anti-inflammatory effect, Robert's geranium may be gargled in the form of tea to treat inflammation in the mouth and throat. It is also used to lessen inflammation of the gastrointestinal tract and diarrhea and to treat lingering wounds, eczema and insect bites.

Tea

The tea is made by pouring about 200 ml of boiling water over 1 to 2 teaspoonsful of the herb. After 10 minutes the mixture is strained. Two to four cups of the tea are drunk throughout the day, preferably between meals.

Horse chestnuts

The common horse chestnut (Latin: *Aesculus hippo castanum*) comes from southeast Europe, the Caucasus and the Middle East but is now cultivated throughout Europe as an ornamental plant. It is a fast-growing deciduous tree and can reach a height of 30 meters and an age of 300 years. It is unmentioned by ancient authors, though it grows in the mountains of Greece. It was brought to Central Europe by the Ottomans, who used it as fodder for horses and to treat bronchitis or other respiratory ailments. Unlike chestnuts, they are unpalatable to humans.

The horse chestnut tree is popular in recreational areas like parks and other green urban areas. Owing to its size, it tends to dominate its surroundings and to provide cool shade even on the hottest days. It blossoms from April or May to June, depending on the weather, and the eye-catching candles are white or pink.

Ingredients

The active ingredients are found in the chestnuts. They consist of to 10% of a complex saponin mixture (aescin) and also contain tannins, coumarins and flavanoids.

Effects

Aescin seals the walls of vessels, stopping water seeping into and pooling in tissues and it also improves the blood's circulation and return to the heart. The effect is to strengthen veins and to lessen edema. It also stimulates the flow of lymph, preventing a dreaded blockage, and is anti-inflammatory.

The chestnuts are used only in the form of finished medicinal products available as tablets, capsules, ointments and gels. These ready-to-use preparations usually contain aescin in a standardized dosage as an ingredient. Aescin preparations are used to stimulate lymphatic flow, venous insufficiency, varicose veins, hemorrhoids and nocturnal cramps of the calves and edema.

Aescin preparations should not be used during pregnancy or breast-feeding and should not be given to children. There can be side effects in the form of mild gastrointestinal discomfort or skin reactions.

Dandelion

The dandelion (Latin: *Taraxacum officinale*) is native to Europe and Asia and has spread to temperate areas all round the world. It grows mainly on meadows rich in nutrients, on pastures for livestock, in parks, on fallow land and on the edge of agricultural land. This perennial and robust plant even grows on screes and from the crevices in walls. Its tenacity and vitality are passed on to whoever knows how to use it. Not surprisingly, its reputation has risen in recent years, transforming it from a tiresome weed into a versatile medicinal plant. Its pretty bright yellow flowers can be found in the mountains as well as on the plains below.

The dandelion belongs to the daisy family (Latin: *Asteraceae*) and is a perennial, herbaceous plant with a notable taproot. Depending on the quality of the soil, it can reach a height of 10–30 cm. Its leaves are notable toothed and can be up to 40 cm long and 24 cm wide. The leaves and stems contain a typically milky juice with a bitter taste, protecting it from infections and being eaten.

The yellow composite flowers appear between the start of April and June, and more may appear later in summer. After the period of flowering, the flowers change into 'clocks' made up of feathery Achaea fruit, which the wind is able to waft away. This is why the dandelion is known in German not only as *Löwenzahn* (lion's tooth) but also as *Pusteblume* (puff flower), as children love to blow it and watch the fruit floating away on the breeze.

Ingredients

The leaves and roots usefully contain bitter substances (taraxin), sterols, carotenoids, tannins, flavanoids, inulin, mucliage and potassium.

In naturopathy

It is said to detoxify the lymph and to activate its flow and to stimulate the flow of bile. It protects the liver and even has a slightly positive effect on hepatocellular carcinomas. It is also used in cases of little appetite, indigestion, bloating and a feeling of being too full and has a diuretic effect due to its high potassium content. The dandelion is said to enhance performance, to simulate the metabolism and to relieve weariness. It also helps to lessen the prevalence of acid, so all in all it is an important basic food.

Tea

Pour 150 ml of boiling water over 1 to 2 teaspoonsful of the herb and let it brew for 15 minutes. Dandelion tea is also good for purifying the blood if used together with nettle leaves. In this case, pour 150 ml boiling water over 2 teaspoonsful of the leaf mixture and allow to stand for 10 minutes. Drink a cup of the blend 3 times a day.

Warning

Dandelions should not be used if you have gallstones, obstruction of the bile or are allergic to the daisy family.

Horsetail

The field horsetail (Latin: *Equisetum arvense*) is native to the temperate zones of the northern hemisphere. It often grows in fields, by lanes and among bushes, ranging from lowlands to Alpine regions (2500 m). It is the only surviving member of a family and genus of plants, whose fossils reach back into the Carboniferous period about 390 million years ago, when the earth was covered with forests of horsetails. They are closely related to ferns and bear no flowers.

Otherwise known as snake grass or puzzle grass, it is also known in German as *Scheuerkraut* (scouring herb) because they were used as brushes for scrubbing, owing to their silica content. The Latin name *Equisitum* comes from *equus*, Latin for horse, and *Saeta*, Latin for bristle, since the branches of the box-trunk are as hard as horse-bristles. Medically, use can be made of the field horsetail's leaves, which are gathered from June to September.

Ingredients

Silica
Potassium salts
Flavanoids (quercetin, kaempferol)

Use

It removes surplus lymph from tissues and helps to purify the lymphatic system.
It can be used to rinse the urinary tract, to remove bacteria and to lessen inflammation, also of the kidneys.
It is applied externally on wounds which are healing poorly.

Non-use

It is not used as a flushing therapy for edema due to a limited activity of the heart or kidneys.

Tea

About 150 ml of hot water are poured over 2 to 3 teaspoonsful (2-4 g) of the horsetail then are strained after about 10 minutes. A cup of freshly prepared tea is drunk 3-4 times a day.

Further herbs

Medicinal plants such as goldenrod, birch and stinging nettle are dehydrating and remove excess lymph from tissues.

Bromelain

A blend of enzymes from the stems of pineapples (Latin: *Ananas comosus*), bromelain helps to detoxify the lymph and to stimulate its flow. Scraps of cells and inflammatory substances are broken down, letting them be borne away more easily by the lymph and blood, and proteins causing edema are broken down, lessening edema and water retention. Proteins otherwise stored in the lymph and hindering its flow are likewise broken down, and the blood can circulate better. Bromelain helps the lymphatic system by lessening acidity and removing toxins and slag. It strengthens the immune system and prevents or improves many ailments like sinusitis and a runny nose.

It is available in the form of capsules coated with enteric. For the enzymes to be fully effective, the capsules should be taken 60 to 90 minutes before meals.

Cleansing the gut

Due to the close relationship between the gut and the lymphatic system, the gut flora should be helped to flourish when the lymphatic system has to be purified. Otherwise, if there are toxins, slag and other waste in the gut, some of them will be passed on to the lymph and hinder its flow. Hence, it is a good idea to take a high-quality probiotic, to ensure that the mucous membranes in the gut are able to regenerate, while putrefactive bacteria and fungi are destroyed. A probiotic also strengthens the gut's immune system, helping it in carrying out detoxfication.

Lymphatic cleansing is recommended at the end of colon cleansing or as part of a comprehensive detoxification cure.

Schuessler salts

These are recommended for any kind of detoxification, as they work gently without side effects. The therapy goes back to the homeopathic doctor Wilhelm Schueslller (1821-1898), who ascribed all ailments to an imbalance of minerals in the body's cells and wished to cure them by supplying the minerals in a homeopathic dosage. He also diagnosed ailments by scrutinizing the features of a person's face, to make out which minerals were needed.

Schuessler salts are becoming increasingly popular, since they are effective, have no side effects and are inexpensive. The number of people relying on them as a proven therapy is continuously growing.

Schuessler salts are used as potentiated agents in tablet form and allowed to dissolve slowly in the mouth. The longer they are in contact with the mouth's lining, the greater the effect. They are available in various potencies, D 6 being viewed as the norm. There are 12 Schuessler agents and 15 additional agents. Schuesseler salts can be absorbed directly by body cells, as they do not have to pass through the digestive tract, so the effect can unfold in a subtle but effective way in every cell.

As regards dosage, there are various opinions. Some homeopaths recommend a high dosage, especially at the beginning of treatment., but I recommend taking 1 tablet 3 times daily, except the hot 7. The tablets can be taken dry or be dissolved in hot water beforehand. If they are dissolved, the hot water should be drunk one sip at a time, and the water should be held in the mouth before being swallowed. If you wish to stir the liquid, use a plastic or wooden spoon, not a metal one.

There is no wide agreement about the number of Schuessler salts which can be taken at the same time. Some homeopaths recommend taking only 1, but some see no reason to set a limit. I recommend taking no more than 3.

Schuessler salts for the lymph

Salt no. 7

Magnesium phoshoricum D 6 (magnesium phosphate) has a decisive influence on the fluidity of the lymph, which literally drives on. As already mentioned, the lymphatic system is unlike the bloodstream in having no pump like the heart, so various factors are crucial for the flow. One of these is the ability of the lymphatic vessels to contract, urging the lymph on, and these contractions are supported by magnesium phosphoricum.

This is the only mineral substance with a special effect when dissolved in hot water. To prepare the so-called hot 7, dissolve 7 tablets of magnesium phosphoricum in about 250 ml of boiled hot water, sip the solution, hold it in your mouth for a moment then swallow it, though magnesium phosphoricum can also be sucked like all other minerals, especially if taken for a long time.

Salt no. 10

Natrium sulhporicum D 6 (sodium sulfate) plays an important role in all detoxification organs – including the lymphatic system. The mineral draws water from cells and tissues by osmotic pressure then excretes it, being the most important compound in this respect. It also activates the lymph by stimulating the cells of the lymphatic vessels.

Salt no. 12

Calcium sulfuricum D 12 (calcium sulfate) is a divalent sulfate salt of calcium and has, like all sulfates, a purifying and detoxifying effect. It furthers the rinsing out of metabolic waste products, poisons and pathogens from the lymph. It has also been used successfully to treat purulent inflammation of the lymph nodes, helping the pus to be destroyed and excreted. Due to its strongly stimulating effect on the lymph nodes, calcium sulfate is often more effective in treating purulent inflammation than are other Schuesseler salts. Pus and inflammatory mediators are flushed out of the body much faster. It does not dissolve easily in water so is preferably used in the 12th decimal potency.

Homeopathic remedies for the lymph

The preference for natural treatments with minimal side effects has led more and more people to homeopathy. This was devised by Samuel Hahnemann (1755-1843), whose notions are recorded in his work The Organon of Healing (1st edition 1810). The 1st edition already contains all the essential theories of homeopathy, but the book was later significantly reworked and supplemented.

Unlike allopathy, where usually the symptoms rather than the causes of a disease are treated, homeopathy is about activating the self-healing powers of the body. Moreover, in homeopathy 'similar things are healed through similar things' (Latin: Similia similibus curen tur). In other words, a stimulus is used which otherwise leads to the symptoms to be treated, thus prompting the body to take action

For instance, nettles are able to cause blisters if touched, so if you have blisters already, due to sunburn or other burns, you can treat them by using nettles (Latin: *Urtica urens*) as a homeopathic remedy.

Another example is the kitchen onion (Latin: *Allium cepa*). All housewives know that cutting an onion is not an easy task, as your nose and eyes run, so in homeopathy, the onion is used in a potentiated form to treat a runny cold and watery eyes.

Another example is caffein, found in coffee, black tea, cappuccinos and so on. If any of these is drunk as a nightcap, you are likely to become restless and sleepless and even to have palpitations of the heart. If, on the other hand, you take Coffea (coffein) in the homeopathic form in the evening, you are less likely to become restless, sleepless and jumpy.

In effect, homeopathy is based on the principle that an active substance, which in its purest form causes a certain symptom or set of symptoms in a healthy person and may even be poisonous, helps in its homeopathic form to draw the body's attention to the complaint and to take action. The body's self-healing powers then heal the ailment and its symptoms such as a runny nose.

If you wish to use high potencies from D 30 on, as well as the C potencies and LM or Q potencies, you should consult a competent homeopath, for the higher the potency, the greater the effect. The energy acting on the body and setting the healing in motion is greater. If you prefer to treat yourself, the potencies D 3 to D 12 are more suitable.

A common effect of homeopathic treatment is that ailments worsen a little after the beginning of treatment, as if being aggravated. This often happens in the case of protracted or chronic ailments and is generally a sign that the homeopathic remedy is suited to the ailment, but such a worsening is neither inevitable nor essential. It should also be noted that conventional medicines prescribed by a physician should never be discontinued or replaced by homeopathic ones.

Nonetheless, nearly all homeopathic remedies can be combined with conventional medicine, as there are rarely any harmful interactions. On the contrary, a combination of conventional and homeopathic remedies can often be very useful. If there is no improvement after 14 days of treatment with a certain homeopathic remedy, there is a need for a different homeopathic remedy.

The treatment should be continued only till health returns, for if you overdo it, the symptoms may return. Homeopathic remedies should be taken at least half an hour before a meal or two hours after one, not at the same time, and toothpastes with peppermint or menthol should be avoided during treatment. Homeopaths may recommend some toothpastes without menthol for you.

During treatment, you should avoid peppermint sweets, mint tea, licorice and chewing gum apart from chewing gum without menthol or peppermint oil. You should also avoid sharp spices, garlic, alcohol, nicotine and cola. If you cannot avoid them, there should be an ample interval of about two hours between consumption and the use of homeopathic remedies.

You should also avoid herbal liqueurs and brandy as well as drinks with quinine, such as Schweppes and take globuli or tablets only with a wooden or plastic spoon, not a metal one, as they may otherwise interact with the metal.

Globules, tablets and dilutions should always be kept in a dry, cool place, never in the refrigerator or near electrical gadgets, and globuli and tablets should be dissolved in the mouth slowly for better absorption. Tablets can also be placed in the pouch of the cheek or dissolved in warm water to be drunk in small sips. Before being swallowed, the liquid should be held in the mouth for a while.

Here are some homeopathic remedies for detoxifying the lymph. The treatment should be chosen according to with the symptoms.

Phytolacca

Phytolacca americana, the American blackberry, belongs to the family of pokeweed plants (Latin: *Phytolaccacae*). A perennial, herbaceous plant reaching a height of 1-3 meters, it is native in North America but has spread over most of the world. It has a strong homeopathic effect on the lymphatic system, especially on the lymph nodes round the neck and chest, and is used in treating influenza, sore throat, tonsils, and throat and parotid glands. If there is difficulty in breastfeeding, Phytolacca stimulates the flow of milk, and inflamed nipples heal faster. Here are the symptoms for taking it.

Symptoms

You tend to be indifferent, listless, irritable and restless. Your mammary glands are hard and swollen, and breastfeeding is painful. There is great pain in your head and back, and pain in your muscles and joints. You find swallowing hard, as your throat is a deep red and burns, and you have recurring angina. Your condition may be improved by cold drinks, rest, fresh air and dry weather. Wet and cold weather, hot drinks, exertion and movement are likely to worsen it.

Conium

The spotted hemlock (Latin: *Conium maculatum*) belongs to the family of the umbelliferae (Latin: *Apiaceae*) and is a biennial herbaceous plant reaching a height of 1-2 meters. It typically smells like mouse urine and is found throughout Europe and in parts of Asia and North Africa. In America and New Zealand, it has become naturalized.

It grows in fields and on paths, rubbish dumps and fallow land and is one of the most poisonous species of umbelliferous plants. A potion from its fruits or roots was used in antiquity to put offenders like Socrates to death. As a medicine, hemlock is nowadays used only in homeopathic doses.

In homeopathy, it is used to treat indigestion and swelling of the lymph nodes, weakness, depression, fatigue and impotence. It also lessens physical and mental paralysis and inner numbness and is commonly used to treat lumps in the female breast and enlargement of the prostate. It improves dizziness, dry cough, heartburn and acidic regurgitation.

Symptoms

Your are mentally lethargic, forgetful, listless and weary in body and mind and sometimes hysterical and stubborn, inclined to weep. You have spells of dizziness and overreact to light. Your skin is yellowish and keratinized. You have night sweats but feel better when in the dark or exercising. You feel worse at night after alcohol or sexual abstinence and are unable to tolerate milk.

Clematis

Clematis recta or the upright clematis belongs to the buttercup family (Latin: *Ranuncu laceae*). As implied by its name, it differs from other species of clematis in growing upright without climbing. Endangered, perennial and herbaceous, it reaches a height of 50-150 cm and grows in bush forests and clearings from Central, Eastern and Southern Europe to the Caucasus. The homeopathic remedy is made from stems together with their flowers and leaves, which are harvested at the beginning of flowering.

Clematis has a strong effect on lymph nodes, even those hardened and swollen, and this applies especially to the lymph nodes of the groin. Other regions affected are the urinary tract, the male and female reproductive organs and all glands such as the prostate. It can heal hardened testicles and mammary glands, improve the retention of urine and inflammation of the bladder and be used to treat itchy rashes on the skin or sleep disorders.

Symptoms

You are often sad, annoyed, weary, dissatisfied, grumpy or contrite or tend to have headaches, especially in the evening. Your sleep is very restless, often accompanied by night sweats, and you have itchy rashes or burning of the urethra. Your symptoms are improved by fresh air and are worsened by physical contact, movement, bed warmth, cold weather and night.

Scrophularia

Scrophularia nodosa, otherwise known as figwort, woodland figwort and common figwort, belongs to the family of figworts (Latin: *Scrophulariaceae*). It is a herbaceous perennial, reaches a height of 50-100 cm and grows in moist areas in forests, on forest verges, among bushes and on riverbanks, needing only medium quality soil. Common figwort is found throughout Europe and western Asia to the Caucasus and western Siberia and has been introduced to North America.

Scrophularia is used in homeopathy for all ailments of the lymphatic system, like weakness of the system and the hardening and swelling of lymph nodes, which it is mostly able to normalize. It is also used to treat immune deficiency, colds, chronic bronchitis, tonsillitis and infections of the throat and middle ear. It can be applied to the gastrointestinal tract, as it improves indigestion and cramps there, and is effective in treating skin itchy for no clear reason, wounds inflamed and slow to heal, eczema and neurodermatitis.

Symptoms

You feel discouraged or depressed, drowsy or dizzy, are quickly exhausted and averse to light, and you often have headaches in the morning. You may also have a dry cold with sneezing. You feel better in a warm room, worse in chilly air or after eating or when lying on your right side.

General detoxification

A detoxification cure should aim at not only supporting and stimulating the organs of detoxification but also at strengthening and detoxifying the body as a whole. General measures undertaken for this should aim at stimulating the metabolism, to ensure that slags, toxins and metabolic end produces are removed from their depots and taken away. Moreover they should stimulate the self-healing powers of the body and the functioning of the immune system.

During treatment it is useful to drink enough flat warm water and herbal tea (about 2.5 l a day), to stay on a healthy diet and to be moderately sportive. If possible, you should avoid alcohol, nicotine and taking medicine, though continual medication should never be abandoned without medical approval, and you should also drink little coffee.

Apart from physical measures such as cupping (see above), you can resort to mainly herbal and homeopathic remedies to remove harmful substances. Manufacturers of homeopathic remedies include DHU, Phoenix, Heel and Wala. Apart from medicines and methods affecting single organs, there are also 'universal remedies' for detoxifying the whole body such as birch coal and algae.

In the field of homeopathy, sulfur has proven to be a 'universal detoxifying agent'. Paracelsus already claimed in the 1500s that sulfur consumes all pathogens, owing to the fire within it. It stimulates the metabolism strongly and is taken preferably in the potency D 12. Further agents for general detoxification are *Arsenicum album* (white arsenic) and antimony in the same potency. The combination agents Derivatio from the firm Pflüger, and Entoxin from the firm Spenglersan, are likewise popular.

An effusion therapy also involves optimizing the balance of acids and alkalies. Due to unhealthy life styles and nutrition, most people are acidified, and the pH value of the urine can easily be found by using indicator paper or strips, available in all pharmacies. For reliable results, you should measure the pH value of the urine several times a day over a period of at least one week.

To balance acids and alkalies, it is crucial to eat little meat and sausages, as these are acidic, whereas greens and fruits tend to be rich in alkalies (see the relevant chapter on maintaining balance below). During detoxification therapy, there is also a need for revitalizing the immune system. As already mentioned, this can be done by having a sauna, brush massage or moderate exercise, as these purify and strengthen the system. The system is also boosted by vitamins like vitamin C in a high dosage, by trace elements like zinc and by herbs or herbal supplements like sea-buckthorn, coneflower and Siberian ginseng (Latin: *Eleutherococcus*).

Sulfur

In the field of homeopathy, sulfur is used for this purpose. It is also called the 'burning principle of nature', since it acts like a fire which burns all germs and toxins. It should always be included in the treatment of chronic ailments, as it flushes toxins, slags and residues of drugs from the body, letting the body focus on healing itself.

Sulfur applied at the start of a therapy ensures that all pollutants contributing to an ailment are thoroughly removed and that the self-healing powers of the body are activated. The metabolism is fueled and the processes of regeneration are supported. In particular, a liver weakened by too much alcohol, infection and medication is strengthened and relieved. Taking sulfur is basic, like turning over a new leaf.

Symptoms

You feel lugubrious, weary, glum and indifferent or have disorders of the liver and an itchy impure skin. You are always thirsty, your stomach is swollen after eating, and you are unable to withstand much heat. You may also have constipation and hemorrhoids.

Birch

The birch (Latin: Betula pendula), also known as the silver birch, warty birch, European white birch or East Asian white birch, is a species of tree in the birch family (Latin: *Betulaceae*). It is native to central and northern Europe and in southern Europe is found only in the mountains. It is a pioneer tree in being one of the first to settle on bare areas and new sites, and its life is fast and fleeting, as it rises quickly to a height of 15-25 m and reaches an age of no more than 160 years, which is slight for a tree.

The birch has an important role in Germanic folklore. Long before the oak and the linden, it was venerated as holy, and people would pick a maypole out of the forest and set it up on a village square. It was a way to bring the awakening spring and nature into the village, as is done even today. The birch is the epitome of spring and merrymaking, of new beginnings and reawakening life, and in this sense it restores our vigor, expelling slags and poisons from our limbs, reviving our bodies and releasing new powers.

Especially in spring and fall, birch leaves are a suitable treatment in the form of tea, juice or elixir. They cleanse, purify and detoxify the body and wash deposits, acids and other noxious substances away and stimulate the kidneys. In general, the birch stands for all processes of flow and renewal so is an effective antidote for weariness and weakness. Birch oil can also be applied to the outside of the body, to relax and strengthen it. The beneficial properties of birch leaves are due mainly to flavonoids as well as to essential oils, saponins, tannins, bitter substances and vitamin C.

The easiest way to enjoy these effects is to drink birch-leaf tea, but an elixir made by gently cooking the young birch leaves and preserving them with sugar is likewise effective.

Ginger

Ginger (Latin: *Zingiber officinale*) is a perennial herb reaching a height of 50-150 or more centimeters and looks like a reed but belongs to the ginger family. It grows in the tropics and sub-tropics and is cultivated for instance in India, Sri Lanka, Indonesia, Vietnam, China, Japan and Nigeria. The active ingredients are in the rhizome and include gingerol and essential oils like zingiberen and curcumen.

Ginger tastes very hot and warms the tuber from inside, but the warming effect benefits us not only on cold wintry days but in general by stimulating the digestive system, the circulation and the metabolism. It increases the body's production of heat and stimulates the organism to release toxins.

Regular consumption of ginger also helps to keep the liver healthy and increases its performance. As it also strengthens the immune system, regular cups of ginger tea are effective against colds. It also stimulates the production of gastric juice and bile and prevents travel sickness. Just 5 g of ginger root a day is enough for it to have a detoxifying effect.

To make the tea, peel a piece of ginger root about two centimeters thick, slice it, pour hot water over the slices then let the tea steep for 5 minutes. You can drink the tea pure, but a tea made from ginger root, nettle leaves and lemon juice is especially cleansing. Ginger roots also taste delicious in green tea, and the blend of the two doubles the detoxifying effect. Ginger tastes fine with other teas too, like tea from lemongrass

Ginger is often used in fruit juice such as orange juice or grapefruit juice and to enrich popular smoothies. There are recipes for carrot-ginger-smoothies, cucumber-ginger smoothies and beetroot mango-ginger smoothies. Indeed, there are no limits to individual creativity. Ginger is also used as an ingredient in sauces and soups, especially in recipes from Asia. Potato ginger soups are very popular, and ginger is often added to coconut and pumpkin soups, carrot and orange soups, lentil soups and Asian noodles. It is also often used in spicy curry dishes and some dishes with greens or fruit like pears.

Food as a remedy

Fruits and greens contain substances important for the health of our bodies and for detoxifying and purifying the organism. Food is healthy if it has plenty of so-called secondary plant ingredients, and these very effective boons from nature sustain our health in various ways:

Caratonoids in carrots for instance ensure our well being, and the same is true of polyphenols in grapes, sulphites in garlic and terpenes in citrus fruits. Whoever regularly consumes these bio-active substances has more body energy and lessens the risk of developing cancer, diabetes, cardiovascular diseases and simple colds.

Fresh greens and fruit contain not only secondary plant ingredients but also lots of minerals and vitamins. It is important to take enough vitamins in because our bodies our unable to synthesize them but need them for strengthening the nerves, supporting the immune system and ensuring that our whole metabolism runs smoothly. Greens and fruit are also recommended as an important part of our diet in mostly containing only a few calories.

They nonetheless contain valuable fibers, which have a doubly positive effect. On the one hand, fibers are voluminous and thereby stimulate a healthily natural function of the gut and digestion and on the other hand they lessen the uptake and increase the excretion of toxins. Fruits and green also contain a lot of alkalies so help our bodies not to have an excess of acid.

Greens & fruit

These should be bought as fresh as possible and be prepared straightaway. The amounts of vitamins and minerals in greens and fruits depends on their quality and freshness, so it is good to check these before buying. Buy greens and fruit which are in season and favor domestic products. After all, transporting greens and fruit from far overseas may take weeks, so this is likely to affect their quality and they may have been subjected to conservatives.

Moreover, greens and fruit taste best when in season. Asparagus is dehydrating and rejuvenating in spring, strawberries and cherries are refreshing in summer; apples and quinces are tasty in fall and strengthen the immune system and prepare the body for the coming of winter, when typical winter greens like Brussels sprouts are a pleasant change.

If the greens and fruit added to your shopping bag are organically grown, you have done everything properly. Growing greens and fruit organically adds little to the chemical burden placed upon our environment, and the produce contains a greater portion of vitamins and minerals.

The fivefold rule

The so-called fivefold rule can easily be integrated into your everyday life. It only means that you should eat at least five helpings (one being a handful) of greens and fruit every day for the sake of your health and metabolism. This can be done without any effort, as the five portions can easily be made part of the main meals. Greens and fruit are also healthy in snacks in between. Greens and fruit are low in calories and supply our bodies with important materials, so they play an important role in preventing ailments due to poor food.

The food pyramid

The so-called food pyramid serves to ensure a healthy and balanced diet. The pyramid is based on water, drunk throughout the day. All organs need water for their manifold tasks, so the metabolism can fulfill its many tasks only if enough water is available. If we drink too little, it hinders the circulation of the blood, then circulatory problems and even constant muddle ensue.

The second tier of the pyramid is made up of greens and fruit, which provide us with vitamins, minerals, trace elements and important secondary phytonutrients. We thereby acquire fibers without being burdened with calories. 5-10 servings of greens and fruit a day are recommended.

The higher tiers of the pyramid become increasing narrow. The third tier is made up of carbohydrates, which provide us with energy. It is best to eat whole grain cereals, as they are rich in fibers, minerals and nutrients.

The fourth tier of the pyramid is made up of milk and dairy products like yogurt and cheese, which provide us with valuable protein and also with calcium for a strong skeleton. 3-6 servings a day are recommended.

The fifth tier is made up of meat and fish, to be eaten only moderately. Given a choice between them, choose fish, as it has unsaturated fatty acids, which our bodies are unable to produce for themselves. We likewise need oils and fats for their high content of unsaturated fatty acids, but they are to be taken sparingly, owing to their high calorie content. Oils and fats also ensure that vitamins soluble in fat are absorbed, but when buying oils and fats, you should favor high-quality vegetable oils rich in unsaturated fatty acids.

The sweet seducers such as chocolate and ice cream should be reserved for special occasions, not be consumed daily. The same applies to snacks like chips and flips as well as sweet drinks.

Breakfast – the main meal

As part of a healthy and energizing diet, breakfast is the most important meal of the day and crucial for getting off to a good start. In the morning you should treat yourself to a lavish and generous breakfast, to provide you with nutrients for the day ahead. The old rule of eating like an emperor in the morning is not old fashioned but as up to date as ever. Before breakfast you should start with a small ceremony: first drink a big glass of lukewarm water with some freshly squeezed lemon juice., to which you may also add ginger or nettles. Lukewarm water is especially easy for the body to cope with, and the addition of lemon, ginger and nettles gets your metabolism moving and frees the body of troublesome waste products which have accumulated overnight.

Fresh fruit

An ideal way to begin the day is to eat plenty of fresh fruit. Good fruit tastes best in the morning and is an ideal complement to muesli and porridge. By enjoying fresh fruit in the morning, you brace yourself for the day ahead right from the start.

Carbohydrates

An ideal breakfast is also made up of complex carbohydrates from whole grain cereals such as oatmeal, rye and spelt flakes, tigernuts, rice, millet, amaranth or quinoa. According to taste, you can make muesli from cereals flakes (like oats, spelt, tigernuts, rice or millet) or make warm or cold porridge from whole grain rice, buckwheat or millet.

Whereas most kinds of cereals used for breakfast muesli produce acid on being metabolized, tigernuts are a welcome exception in producing alkalies, so by eating them in the morning you help to establish a healthy ratio of alkalies and acids.

The tigernut, also called chufa, is a species of plant belonging to the genus of Cyprus grasses native to lands round the Mediterranean. Apart from the basic ingredients, more than 25% of a tigernut is made up of valuable unsaturated acids. The abundant fibers sate hunger for a long time and also prevent a drop of the level of blood sugar. All in all, it is worthwhile to get to know the tigernut better and to incorporate it regularly into your diet.

Office hours

You can also eat healthily in the office too. You do not always have to buy sandwiches and sweet rolls from the kiosk on the corner. Take plenty of fruit and vegetables to work for your breaks and also snack on almonds, olives and dried fruit. Instead of relying only on coffee as a pick-me-up, you can try a blend of lettuce in water and also take a chance to stretch your limbs. In the canteen, the ideal ingredients are lettuce, greens in general and potatoes rather than meat, noodles and eggs.

Variety

Variety is the spice of life and of good food. By varying your diet, you ensure that you have enough vitamins, minerals and trace elements and avoid pollutants, present in greater amounts in certain foods. Every food has its own range of valuable ingredients, so a balanced diet is always varied, to cover the range. It is also a delight to have something different and adds to our appreciation of the taste.

A healthy natural diet

In the course of our lives, most of us get used to processed foods, ready meals, sweets, snacks and, of course, alcohol and sweetened drinks. Without thinking too much about the consequences, we start the day with a croissant dripping with fat, followed by a cappuccino. In the lunch break, we have French fries with mayonnaise, then in the afternoon cake with coffee, to revive our flagging spirits. Such is our way of life, but why treat or abuse your body in this way? Why care so little about your own health?

We take plenty of care of our cars, clothes, homes and budgets. We clean our homes in spring and fall, use the best cleaning agents and polishes and we pay attention to every stain and scratch, to ensure that our furniture and carpets remain spic and span as long as possible. We go regularly to the hairdresser, to the nail salon and pamper our skin, our envelope, with various vials, masks, creams and serums.

Why then do we neglect our bodies so criminally, cramming it with harmful and unhealthy food? Is due to carelessness, comfort, habit or lack of awareness? It may be a combination of all these. It may also be due to the fact that neglected hair or fingernails are immediately noticeable, whereas our bodies say nothing and put up with neglect for too long, till the first signs of discomfort or even disease become evident.

But better late than never! We may still have time to switch to a healthy diet and way of life. Where there is a will, there is also a way. Just as we get used to fast food and ready meals, we can also get used to healthy food and do so amazingly fast.

We are what we eat

This saying from the French gastronome Brillat-Savarin is not a hackneyed phrase but a telling truth. The weight of our own bodies, which we have to bear, reflects not only a good or bad metabolism, as we often explain apologetically, but also our daily dietary habits, and if our skin looks bad or pale, this may be due to not only 'bad' genes but also an unhealthy diet or even smoking. Likewise the widening gaps in the sieves of our memories may be due as much to more alcohol as to more years behind us.

Besides, one pint of beer at lunchtime and a glass of red wine in the evening add up in the course of time. We are always quick to attribute our condition to genetic inheritance or other factors, but ailments and mood disorders seldom occur without good reason and are more often home-made than due to fate. If we are plump, it is not something which has happened to us overnight but is due to years of overeating, especially the wrong food. We all too easily forget this. Our habits of eating often reflect our values and our general way of life:

A vegetarian is less likely to abstain from meat for health reasons than for ethical reasons; a conservationist buys his food in a health food store; and a philanthropist pays attention to fair-trade coffee. Hence our habits of eating express our identities and values. Different cultures and different societies have their own eating habits. The cow is holy to the Hindu, whereas Koreans are willing to eat dogs. As for the French, they have nothing against frogs' thighs, pig's gonads and similar tidbits.

Nutrition today

As a matter of fact, I have quite a good diet, you may be inclined to say. But is this really true if you think about it? In the morning you cheer yourself up with a cup of coffee then eat a chocolate bar in the lunch break. In the afternoon, you have cake with auntie's coffee then get over the stress of work with a cigarette. In the evening you have a beer before going to bed. And who would object to some peanuts on the settee in front of the television?

Lunch is ready made, but at least the packaging promises a tasty meal without many calories, and the drink may be sugary but also full of vitamins. Food is plentifully available so is eaten to any extent. Whereas food used to be scarce, and meat ended up only as roast on the Sunday table, and chocolate and cakes were reserved for feast days, even unhealthy foods such as meat and sweets are no longer viewed as something special but are served as daily treats.

But though food is available in more than enough quantity, the quality is often lacking. There are too few vitamins and minerals, but as long as the food is cheap and plentiful, it is bought and eaten. If you want to buy healthy, untreated food, you may have to visit the hidden health-food shop round the corner. Shiny apples in supermarkets may be a feast for the eyes, but they are so often treated with pesticides that it would hardly be overdoing it to label them with a skull and crossbones. They look good, but vitamins and minerals are hard to find in this designer fruit.

Leaching of the soil decreases the mineral content and increases pollution from heavy metals, which find their way from the soil into our food. The situation is hardly better if you choose to dine out. Roast pork and beef fillet are on the menu, and cakes are colorfully on show just behind the counter, so if you ask for organic food, you may be viewed as an alien posing an odd question.

Nutrition as it used to be

Our forebears were well adapted to their environments and thus to their natural diets. Already in the Bible (Genesis 1, 29-31), the '**seeds and fruits**' are assigned to mankind as a privilege and suitable source of nourishment. In many ways, we are more like our forebears in the stone age than we like to think. Our bodies are still adapted to meager plant food, gathered by hand in the course of long migrations. Meat was an exception rather than the rule, as the animals had to be hunted, killed and carried away, carved up and properly prepared.

Our forebears in the stone age had no modern concoctions such as sweets and cakes and they fed mainly on plants, seeds, nuts, mushrooms, fruit, roots and other parts of plants. In bad times, when there was little or no food available, the body had to live off its stores of fat, which is why it made sense to put on weight in the first place. In some respects, our inherited inclinations and the processes in our bodies still rely on this kind of nutrition.

Training taste

What we like is determined largely by our upbringing and habits. Even in the womb, we are affected by the smell and taste of the food consumed by our mothers. This benefits the food industry, which accustoms our palates to all kinds of additives and flavor enhancers, so we really become obsessed with finished products and buy them again and again.

Our taste-buds get used to all kinds of flavorings and become dissatisfied with the milder taste of natural foods, but luckily, just as we can get used to enhanced flavors, we can also get used to the natural level of flavoring again. We should try gradually to reacquire a taste for unadulterated food and to appreciate the taste of unprocessed food.

Foods to be avoided

To strengthen and detoxify the body, it is not enough to eat a lot of greens and fruit, even though these are part of a healthy diet. It is equally important to refrain from indulging in foods which poison our bodies. These include all sugary products like chocolate, ice-cream, cakes, candies, chocolates and so on. Sugar not only poisons and weakens the body but also extracts valuable vitamins and minerals from it. Besides, overeating, eating too much meat and all kinds of ready-made meals hardly lead to good health.

Meals ready-made

We are continually tempted to turn to ready-made food and finished products for the sake of saving time. The deliciously-looking food straight from the freezer or shelf is often a feast for the eyes but does not have as much to offer in terms of nutritional value. Such foods have been greatly modified by chemical, mechanical or thermal processing, till they have little of their original composition.

More and more, the processed product becomes unlike the original, and in very few cases is it actually improved in the process. Heat for instance removes vitamins, minerals and fibers, which may otherwise be adequately present.

Meat – the red risk

Especially red meat like beef, pork, lamb and goat meat has been frowned upon by nutritionists and health-conscious people for a long time, as it can severely harm your health and shorten your life. Anyone who eats a lot of red meat and products made from it, like sausages, is 1.3 times more likely to die young than is someone who never eats it, other things being equal. The main causes of death in such cases are heart attacks and cancer, due in turn to the carcinogenic substances made by the roasting of red meat and to the high content of saturated fatty acids.

Even a limited consumption of red meat, such as 150 g daily, is enough to shorten your life, so the amount is secondary. White meat like chicken or turkey is not as harmful, but considering the conditions under which these birds are kept, there are also ethical aspects. They are also environmental ones, for 15-25 % of the water used globally flows into livestock, who then emit nearly 20% of greenhouses houses, which is more than is emitted even by traffic.

Killer fats

Trans-fatty acids present a very special danger within the group of fats and, from a nutritional point of view, are among the undesirable parts of our diet. But what does the term trans-fatty acid actually mean? The 'trans' stands for transfigured fatty-acid, and what are transfigured are the carbon double bonds. Trans-fatty acids are especially common in industrially produced foods, where they are due to the hardening of vegetable oils. For instance they are abundant in French fries, potato chips and various fats for baking and frying. They are most concentrated in puff pastry, cooking oil and instant soups.

Good & bad carbohydrates

A good way to assess carbohydrates is to draw a line between the good and the bad by using the so-called Glyx principle. The glycemic index (abbreviated to GI) is a measure for determining the effect of a food containing carbohydrates on the blood sugar level. The glyx alludes to the increase in blood sugar after eating and thus also to the body's insulin reaction. More technically, it is defined as the relative area under the 2-hour blood sugar curve after taking 50 grams of carbohydrates. The effect of glucose on blood pressure is used as a reference value.

High GI foods cause a sharp increase in blood sugar levels, which then cause a great amount of insulin to be released. Proponents of the glyx principle suspect that as a results of eating foods with a high GI, there is an under-supply of glucose about 2-4 hours after eating them. This leads to a feeling of hunger and to eating food which swiftly increases the amount of blood sugar, so in effect there is a vicious circle and a steady increase in body mass.

According to this line of thought, it is important to switch to carbohydrates with a low GI for the sake of staying slim. The so-called good carbohydrates have a GI of less than 50 and cause the blood-sugar level to rise only slowly, so they are followed by no sudden hunger. Good carbohydrates are carbohydrates with enough fiber. They are found in foods like whole grains, greens and fruit, so these can be eaten liberally.

The bad carbohydrates include processed cereal products like white bread, peeled rice and all kinds of sweets, so of course they should be generally avoided. They are made up of simple sugars, known as monosaccharides, which quickly boost insulin levels and have a GI index above 50. There are now several diets which attach importance to the glyx principle, like the Montignac method, the glyx diet and the logi method.

Critics of the glyx principle rightly claim that the knowledge is not new but only old wine in new bottles. Indeed, it has been recommended for a long time that for the sake of good nutrition and loss of weight we should eat whole grains and a lot of greens and fruit, while avoiding sweets and white-flour products.

The German Society for Nutrition dismisses the glyx principle on the grounds that our weight is determined by the overall balance of energy in our bodies and that the GI depends on a person's individual metabolism, so a given amount of carbohydrates does not have the same effect on the insulin level of one person as it does on the insulin level of another. Moreover, adding up the GIs of each part of a meal may not be enough, especially as the GI of a foodstuff changes when the food is processed.

Acids & alkalies

The modern way of life tends to make our bodies too acidic. They may effectively compensate for a long time and even decades, till finally the efforts come to nothing, and ailments become fully apparent. Whether a food is mainly acidic or not is not always revealed by its taste, for it changes in the course of being processed. Foods which eventually make acids do not always begin with some, so the food does not initially taste sour and may even seem to be neutral or alkaline.

Whoever suspects on eating a bar of chocolate that acids will result in the body? The most which eaters of chocolate tend to fear is the presence of a few calories, so unwittingly they are drawn into the acid trap. If your body is already too acidic, the first and simplest antidote is to choose food which makes alkalies, while avoiding food which makes acids.

Foods which make acids

Animal proteins

The main problem with animal protein apart from the acidity is that too much of it is being eaten, especially in the form of meat and sausage. Whilst a grown-up needs 30-60 g of protein per day (contained in one serving of fish or meat), the actual intake in western industrialized countries is 80-150 g per person per day. These numbers speak for themselves: many people are eating much more protein than is needed so are suffering from the glut. To many people, a meal without meat is unthinkable, and salads and greens are only side dishes.

Factory farming has ethical implications, and meat has more traces of drugs than are found in a home pharmacy. But apart from these considerations, the inevitable result of overeating meat is that our bodies become mercilessly acidified, as protein from animal fat is converted into salts of sulfuric and phosphoric acid, which are strong acids and also acidify the body after being metabolized.

The breakdown of protein also produces uric acid, which is known to play a role in the development of gout, and this acidifying effect varies little from one kind of meat to another. Of course, meat in moderation may be less disastrous, but in that case, it is useful to choose suitable species of animals on organic farms and to cut down on sausages.

Milk products

Milk and dairy products such as cheese and yogurt are converted in the body into slightly acidic end products, thought this drawback is partly offset by their high mineral content. Only raw milk itself has a slightly alkaline effect, but milk commercially available is almost completely pasteurized, and this is chemically modified and acidifying. Raw milk is generally available only to farmers and has the drawback of having possibly more germs. All kinds of cheese are acidifying, though the extent varies according to the kind. Parmesan for instance is more acidifying than cream cheese. Dairy products with a lot of whey, like cottage cheese and yogurt, are not tolerated by people who are already much too acidic.

Cereals

Oats, wheat and barley are healthy but make acids in the body, whether or not we eat them as whole grains, flakes, flour or processed in the form of pasta or biscuits. In this respect there is no difference between wholemeal cereals and refined cereals like husked rice or white bread. Otherwise, whole grains are preferable in having more mineral and vitamin content. Full grain also has enough fiber, which stimulates the digestion and leads to longer satiety.

Moreover, the minerals in the whole grain also supply the body with alkalies, offsetting the acidity to some extent. In general, the smaller a grain of cereal is, the smaller the portion of acidifying protein and the bigger the portion of minerals. The big grains of wheat, rye, oats and rice make much more acid than the small grains of amaranth or quinoa.

Sugary pastries

Sugar and all products containing it like tarts and chocolate create a lot of acid, due the fermentation of sugar. Only unrefined sugars such as brown whole-cane sugar and maple syrup can be classified as neutral foodstuffs, which is why they are preferable to refined ones. The harmful effect of sugar is not limited to its acidifying effect, as it also robs the body of minerals like calcium and vitamins like B 1. Sugar continues to weaken the immune system and can trigger metabolic ailments like diabetes, and every child knows about the harmful effects of sugar on the enamel of the teeth.

Fats and oils

The more refined they are, the more dangerous they are. Especially hardened or refined fats and oils as well as animal fats like lard have a strongly acidifying effect. These fats should be severely restricted, not only because of the calories they contain and their harmful effect on health (refined fats play a role in the development of certain cancers) but also because of the resulting acidifcation. Nonetheless, cold-pressed, gently produced vegetable oils remain neutral in the metabolism and are part of any healthy diet on account of their valuable unsaturated fatty acids.

Additives in foodstuffs such as preservatives, colorants, flavor enhancers and sweeteners are often hidden but no less dangerous acidifiers. Two examples are the flavor enhancer glutamate and the sweetener aspartame.

Determining the body's acidity

This can be done by measuring the pH value of urine, which is easily done at home. Due to the removal of acids and the cleansing done by our bodies during the night, urine is most acidic in the morning then its acidity fluctuates during the day. For the sake of a reliable value, the pH values of the so-called middle jet urine should be determined seven times a day for a week then the mean value be taken as characteristic. A single measurement is unreliable on account of fluctuations.

The seven measurements

These should take place at the following times of day:

Before breakfast (about 7 a.m.)
About two hours after breakfast (about 10 a.m.)
Before lunch (about 12 a.m.)
About three hours after lunch (about 3 p.m.)
Before dinner (about 6 p.m.)
About three hours after dinner (about 9 p.m.)
Before bedtime (about 11 p.m.)

Measuring the pH value

The pH value can easily be found by using so-called indicator sticks or pH paper available in every pharmacy, where you can also get advice. For the sake of accuracy, make sure that the pH paper covers the range of at least pH 4.5-8.4 and displays every 0.2 points. You can either hold the indicator in the middle jet urine or collect the urine in a container and dip the strip into it, making sure that the paper is thoroughly moistened. The result can be read off within 20 seconds.

The pH value of the urine changes very fast and reacts at once to food eaten the day before, which is why it is so important to eat only your usual food during the period of measurement. Certain medications such as acetylsalicylic acid in aspirin have an acidifying effect, so you should avoid taking any such medicine while measuring the pH values.

Detoxifying the lymph by drinking

The best drink is water, essential for all life. Humans can live for weeks without food and can hunt or gather food for a long time but they can live without fluid intake for only a few days. This is because water is needed as a part of all tissues in our bodies, as a way to transport soluble substances, and as a solvent for nearly all substances in cells. Water also regulates the body's temperature by evaporating from its surface and cooling it down. People in general are about 60% water, though men have slightly more than women, and the young have more than the old.

Drink enough

As a rule of thumb, a grown-up should take in about 2.5 liters a day, though many people take in much less. This is because thirst only appears as a warning signal if the lack of water has already reached an alarming stage. People who drink too little risk suffering from circulatory problems, dizziness, weariness and exhaustion. Besides, if there is too little water, metabolic processes no longer run optimally, so slag may accumulate.

To be sure of drinking enough, you can work out in the morning how much you will need to drink in the course of the day (preferably still water and unsweetened tea) then stick to your plan. This is the only way to be sure that you will take enough in, because if you try to gulp it all down at once, too much water is then released in urine. It is best to drink a glass of water, preferably lukewarm, first thing in the morning, which will also stimulate your digestion, metabolism and detoxification.

Ideally, you should add freshly squeezed lemon juice and/or some fresh ginger or nettle to the water, as this will boost the body and help to detoxify it. It is also a good idea to drink a glass of water about half an hour before every meal and at intervals during the day. This gets the metabolism going, stimulates the kidneys, washes degradation products away and stimulates the combustion of energy.

Fizzy or flat?

Carbon dioxide in fizzy water is an inorganic acid which also acidifies the metabolism, so still water is better. Besides, if you drink still water, you can gulp down generous amounts without belching in high society or bloating like a zeppelin.

A change of drink

Drinking nothing but mineral water may seem rather monotonous after awhile, so feel free to try various concoctions. Even mineral waters differ from one another, and unsweetened herbal teas are tasty and good for the health. Besides, most of them bias you towards alkalies and help to detoxify and purify your body, letting you feel healthier and livelier.

Green Tea

This is welcome treat from the far east and becoming popular worldwide. Unlike the leaves of black tea, the leaves of green tea are hardly fermented or not at all, so vitamins and minerals are still available for the person savoring it. Like coffee, it contains caffeine, but unlike the caffeine in coffee, it is bound partly to tannin, which stimulates the nervous system gradually, not speeding the circulation up at once.

Green tea also stimulates the metabolism, increasing the excretion of toxins. Green tea also contains large amounts of bitter substances which, if taken regularly, can modify the sensation of taste, making sweet foods taste less pleasant and bitter foods more pleasant. Moreover, bitter substances are good for the liver and further its detoxifying activity. By activating detoxification and the metabolism, it provides the body with fresh energy.

Juices rich in vitamins

You can improve your health fairly easily by regularly drinking fruit and vegetable juices. It is best to drink juices freshly squeezed, as these contain the greatest amounts of vitamins, minerals and fiber. As concentrates, juices are often thermally treated or filtered, whereby they lose a significant portion of the valuable ingredients. And do not be fooled by the sham '**nectar**', which often contains up to 20% sugar and little fruit. Take a little time to study the labels before buying any. It is also a good idea to dilute the juices, as this lessens the calorie-load while still giving you an energizing drink.

Sleep & detoxification

Sleeping enough is a very effective way to regenerate and detoxify the body. This is because during sleep the metabolism works at full speed. The body is not preoccupied with other tasks so can dedicate itself to detoxification and purification. Moreover the body needs rest and relaxation to regenerate itself and its organs properly. During sleep, new cells are formed, existing cells are improved and damaged cells are mended or eliminated. Free radicals able to cause ailments are destroyed during sleep, as are all kind of pathogens such as viruses, bacteria and fungi.

It is not for nothing that we talk of having a healthy sleep, as a restful sleep awakens the spirits again and rejuvenates all bodily functions. This regeneration takes place mainly in the first half of the night, in the so-called phase of deep sleep between 11 in the evening and 3 in the morning.

The optimal period of sleep varies from person to person, but on average a person needs seven to eight hours. Not enough sleep weakens the body but so does too much sleep or a disturbed day-night rhythm, due for instance to working on shifts. Not only sleep itself but also its quality is crucial. Anyone who sleeps restlessly at night and wakes up feeling jiggered in the morning has not recovered enough, and the immune system is likely to suffer.

The best room temperature for sleeping is 16-19°C. Ideally, the bedroom should not be heated at night, but at need you can grab a thick blanket, thick woolen socks or even a hot water bottle. Before going to bed, open the window wide for a few minutes for the sake of enough fresh air. The humidity in the room should lie between 40-50%.

How to unwind

Stress is a phenomenon of our time. It is found in the workplace, extends into overtime and lessens the time remaining. How many people seldom experience it? Boundless hustle and bustle determine our everyday lives, and the pressure to perform well at work and at home is continually increasing. Like hamsters we are caught in our treadmills.

Even in our free time, we have a whole range of obligations, as our fellow club members call for us and we are expected o socialize. We are loath to miss anything and try to rush off in all directions. At home, we have the Internet and television for stimulation, and the mobile phone keeps on ringing, so we are always on the go. We can be reached by anyone at any time so have no more time for ourselves. Naturally, health and well-being fall by the wayside.

Of course, stress is not the only cause of ailments along with overloading and poisoning the body and soul, but it is the driving force in the development of ailments mental and physical. But what exactly is stress? Stressful situations are marked by over-reliance, helplessness and a loss of control. We feel unable to influence or avoid these situations and unable to cope with them. But this may at times be a subjective assessment, as the situations are really less dangerous or threatening than at first sight. We then put ourselves needlessly under pressure, reacting hectically, cramped and mindlessly.

We also feel stressed, if the fruits of our work are poorly respected and appreciated, but if the stress is sustained, it weakens the mental and physical defenses of the body in various ways. For instance in periods of prolonged stress, the hormone cortisol is increasingly produced in the adrenal cortex and has the unpleasant effect of suppressing the immune system. When the body is continually stressed, it loses its ability to cope with the stress and difficulties, and somewhere along the line, it simply gives up and reacts apathetically.

Continual stress puts the body on red alert – a reaction we have inherited from our forebears in the stone age – and causes the adrenal cortex to produce stress hormones. At the same time, the so-called sympathetic nerve is activated, preparing the body to fight or flee. In general these are called stress reactions. The hormones adrenaline and norepinephrine are freely released, increasing the pulse, blood pressure and blood sugar and quickening breathing.

If the body is continually stressed and there is no longer a balance between tension and relaxation, body and mind fall ill. We have to give them a chance to recharge their batteries and to compensate for the stress by occasionally resting. In a state of deep relaxation, the reset button is pressed, supplying our empty batteries with fresh energy. The body is cleansed, blockages dissolved and we can find inner harmony and peace and restore balance.

Mindfulness

Being mindful means observing all the processes around us with undivided, relaxed attention and absorbing all the details of our surroundings. Instead of losing ourselves in thought, we focus on our awareness and welcome every moment without any ulterior motive. Mindfulness also means not being distracted by anything, because the distracted mind is a stressed mind.

Mindfulness can be practiced by focusing on the here and now and our own awareness or on the simplest things such as breathing. If we learn to be restfully attentive, the quality of our thought pleasantly changes. Negative thoughts lose their power over us, and more and more the little joys of life and the happiness of being alive here and now come to the fore. We feel more relaxed, and stressful situations no longer affect us deeply. Our minds become clearer and we can better understand our habitual thoughts, feelings and reactions.

Practicing mindfulness is meant to help us to observe and accept present thoughts, feelings and bodily sensations, pleasant or unpleasant, without being judgmental. In effect, we look at our own feelings through the eyes of an outsider, then fears, musings, anger and other negative thoughts seem less alarming. Realize how you are feeling and be attentive to everything! The intensity of the experienced moment will make your life richer and happier day by day.

Relaxation techniques

Donkey hiking has plainly become a new trend. Donkeys have an air of deep calmness and serenity, so it is easy to find peace and quiet in their company. Their calmness and serenity spread to the humans near them, letting them feel grounded, centered and balanced. Their friendly and approachable nature invites us to be with them and to linger in the presence of the long-eared.

The communication with donkeys is honest and authentic, even without words. The creature instinctively senses the attitude of a person towards him, and if this is respectful and clear, he accepts the approach. A person called a stubborn ass may indeed owe his mindfulness, strength of character, incorruptibility and reliability to a donkey, for if a donkey is unsure about a situation, he stops and persistently thinks it over. Only if he is finally convinced that all is well does he move on.

Whoever wants to go on a donkey walk should be aware that the pace will be set by the donkey. A donkey is never in a hurry and is always fully alive in the here and now. On average, a donkey covers about three kilometers an hour, so in his company you can forget about forced marches and clocking up mileage. The donkey will grant you a chance to rediscover your slowness. You may then begin to feel that there is really no rush or anything to miss or at least not in the midst of fields and forests in pleasant company.

You learn that the way to your goals is a goal in its own right and that racing and rushing make little sense to a donkey. He will yield to the temptation of fresh greens by the wayside and pause now and then to nibble another shrub on his quest for flavors. Walking with a donkey means pausing to savor the present. Instead of always hurtling into the future, you slow down to relish his company and the landscape. These incorruptible animals meet us with out judging us, which is why they are ideal for therapeutic purposes. Given a chance, accept the adventure of strolling with a donkey.

Yoga

This consists of a set of mental and physical exercises such as asanas, meditation and asceticism with roots in India. The word yoga comes from Sanskrit, the ancient language of India, and means to harness or yoke and was originally applied only to draft animals. It then became applied to humans too in the sense of yoking the body to the soul for the sake of centering and concentration.

Yoga yokes the body, breath and mind, to let them work as a team. Hence, Indian teachings assume that we can maintain our health only by harmonizing body, breath and spirit, which is the goal of nearly all yoga practices. Nonetheless, there are various paths to this goal and they differ markedly from one another.

Though yoga was originally a spiritual discipline, whose ultimate aim to was to heighten awareness, practitioners in Europe and North America often practice only the asanas, the physical exercises, neglecting the religious aspects. Other kinds of yoga emphasize the meditative side of the tradition or parts of it like asceticism, but ways of breathing are always an integral part of the exercises.

When breathing in, we let energy flow into our bodies, and on breathing out, we release tension. Conscious breathing is combined with the asanas (postures), of which there is a strikingly wide variety, quite apart from their variations and preliminary exercises.

Many of the asanas are like the postures of animals so are named after then like the camel, cobra, fish, scorpion, rooster and dog, but there are also other asanas like the plow, bow, hero or tree. The asanas all involve gently stretching though never to the extent of causing pain.

You should not shy away from yoga, whose worldwide popularity continues to grow and provide health benefits. Yoga is a holistic way to safeguard physical, mental and spiritual well-being and helps us to realize that happiness and peace cannot be gained from others but only from ourselves. In effect, it shows us the path to our inner self, challenging us to explore and be aware of our essence.

Mindfulness and awareness are called for and furthered. With continual practice, stress is lessened and body and soul become deeply relaxed, and in daily life, the yogi benefits from having more serenity and patience. Traditionally, yoga is also used to counter fatigue by activating life energy and can help to improve a whole range of ailments, especially cardiovascular ailments, circulatory disorders, headache and backache as well as mental conditions like anxiety, depression and sleep disorders.

The individual exercises train strength, flexibility, coordination and muscular endurance, and the activation of muscles, tendons, ligaments and blood and lymph vessels improves the circulation of the blood. The strengthening of back muscles helps us not to slump at a desk. Yoga also has a soothing and balancing effect so may counter the consequences of stress.

Breathing exercises and meditation are likewise used to reach inner peace, but if you decide to take up yoga, you should by no means do it only alone at home in a quiet room and learn it only from books. If you fail to do the complicated exercises properly, you may end up by doing yourself a mischief. You should rather learn yoga from a qualified teacher, which is possible at yoga schools, in gyms and at community colleges.

There are many styles of yoga but all are branches of hatha yoga, which is the kind practiced most widely in the west and is the kind generally meant if yoga is mentioned. The individual exercises are often strung together in series with harmonious transitions between them as in the case of the salutation to the sun (*sūrya namaskār*).

Breathing is of special importance here, because the sequences of movements can be done effectively only with suitable breathing. Other popular styles of yoga include kundalini, kriya and bikram yoga. All in all, yoga is one of the most effective means of relaxation ever devised. Slow and focused movements and controlled breathing quieten the central nervous system, enhancing balance and relaxation.

Detox yoga

Besides being generally good for the health, some yoga exercises also specifically further the detoxification of body and soul. Especially twisting movements and bending forward have a purifying effect like an inner massage. Their cleansing effect furthers the functioning of the organs involved in detoxification like the liver, intestine and kidneys, letting them achieve their aims more fully.

Special exercises, such as the lord of the fishes posture (*matsyendrāsana*) or the pliers posture (*paścimottānāsana)* twist or bend the body, squeezing slag and toxins out of the inner organs while enriching them with fresh oxygen. The metabolism and flow of blood are optimized and digestion is stimulated, so we are able to rid ourselves of pollutants and waste products.

Even so-called flows or flowing movements, in which one exercise blends into the next, further the circulation of the blood and thereby detoxification. Other exercises good for this purpose are the shoulder stand, the crocodile and the frog. These exercises not only massage and stimulate the detoxification organs but also release negative thoughts, so are detoxifying in the psychological sense too and they further self-healing powers.

Movements involving twisting the spine, as in the sequence known as the eight movements of the spine, also ensure a thorough detoxification and strengthening of the body. *Kapalabhati* breathing, a kind of snorting often used in yoga, has likewise a strong cleansing and detoxifying effect.

Meditation

'The mind must be empty to see clearly.'

(Jiddu Krishnamurti, 1895-1986, an Indian philosopher and author)

Often our thoughts revolve and refuse to settle down, being overwhelmed by stress, anger and anxiety. However hard we try, we find it hard to shrug off the abundant ballast in our brains. Meditation can help to empty the mind and to let go. With regular practice, we can stop the roundabout of thoughts and stay in the here and now.

With all our senses, we are then involved in the present moment and the worries of everyday life no longer matter. Through meditation, can can learn to control our thoughts instead of letting our thoughts control us. Our minds becomes clearer, our bodies and souls regain their balance and we find our centers of gravity again. We have a sense of inner peace, and body and soul relax and feel at ease.

By meditating, we can break our dubious habits and realize why we act in certain ways and thereby become wiser. If we meditate regularly, we feel calmer, more harmonious, happier, more peaceful and stronger inside.

The word *meditation* comes from the Latin words *meditatio* (attention to the middle) and *medius* (median) and describes a spiritual practice shared by many religions and cultures. The aim is to calm the mind down and to concentrate it by practicing mindfulness. The desired states of consciousness are often described by terms such as stillness, emptiness, being at one with ourselves, being here and now and free from thoughts.

In eastern cultures, meditation is thought to be a basic exercise for intensifying awareness, so as a spiritual practice it has become part of various religious, psychological and ethical teachings. In western countries, it is often practiced outside the framework of religion for the sake of general well-being, stress-relief and psychotherapy. In fact, there are countless kinds of meditation techniques, differing according to their religious origins. Especially in Hinduism, Buddhism and Taoism, meditation has a similar meaning to prayer in Christianity.

Apart from traditional techniques of meditation, many kinds inspired by teachings in the far east and adapted to western needs have been offered to the west, especially since the 1970s. But all kinds share the aim of bringing about a state of awareness differing from the everyday state in being focused wholly on the present. There are no glances back at the past in the form of memories or at the future in the form of plans or fears. The aim is to achieve a state of awareness which is clear and alert but also extremely relaxed.

In general a line is drawn between passive and active meditation. The former is practiced while sitting still, and the latter involves physical exercise, attentive action or even loud recitation. Mostly, the term meditation is applied to the former,, as seen in paintings of the meditating Buddha, whereas the latter includes tantra, yoga and the martial arts.

In meditation, you focus your mind on just one thing, instead of moving from one thing to another, as we do in our daily lives. The focal point may be a word like Om – So-Ham – Ham, which even has a reassuring sound. The aim is to empty your mind of all other thoughts and, if any return, to refocus on the chosen sound. It is also important to have a comfortable posture, letting you sit still for 20-60 minutes, as your periods of meditation become longer.

Tai chi

Otherwise known as Chinese shadow boxing, this began as a martial art in the Chinese empire. More recently, the martial side of it has waned, and tai chi is becoming a popular sport which helps you to meditate and to develop your personality. The soft and flowing movements put the body into a state of deep relaxation and further peace and equanimity.

Qi gong

This is an ancient Chinese way to relax and it relieves stress, awakens vitality and furthers serenity. The movements are slow, meditative and fluid and able to resolve blockages and tension as well as to coordinate breathing and movement. It combines concentration, meditation and movement for the cultivation of body and mind and also includes breathing exercises.

The name qu gon is relatively new, though some of the exercises have been part of Chinese culture for well over a thousand years. Qi gong means literally energy work and refers to exercises which are meant to cultivate the qi or life force, though as well as meaning work, gong also means practice or task, depending on context. The various exercises serve to enrich and harmonize the qi (pronounced chi), which stands for the moving and vital principle of not only the body but also the world.

The practice of qi gong is meant to strengthen the life energy and thereby to prolong life and to help to maintain a healthy mental state. The individual exercises are said to take in energy from the surroundings and to ease its flow, thereby benefiting body and mind, and range from stretching and breathing to running. The three most common systems are the Eight Brocade Exercises, the Game of the Five Animals, and the Six Healing Lutes.

The Eight Brocade Exercises are the most popular in being very easy to learn and are taught in qi gong schools. The body becomes more robust, the mind and breathing lbenefit, joints are protected and muscles and tendons are gently stretched.

The Game of the Five Animals consists in imitating the movements of deer, monkeys, bears, cranes and tigers are imitated. For each animal, there are several exercises which support and nourish the flow of energy to the organs, whereby the powers and instincts of these animals are acquired.

The Six Healing Sounds are meant to penetrate the body in the form of vibrations, to stimulate regions otherwise inaccessible.

Music, baths & scents

Music

What could be lovelier after a long and hard day at work than to hear the sounds of relaxing music. Healing sounds relax the body and mind and grant inner peace and harmony. They give us a chance to ignore unpleasant stimuli, to withdraw from everyday life, to empty ourselves of worries and to regain our balance. Sounds float through the room, inviting us to join them, so begin the evening with a wellness CD, as you surely deserve.

Sounds from nature are especially harmonious and reassuring like the hovering of the wind, the surging of the sea, the burbling of a stream, the twittering of birds or the singing of whales. Underscored perhaps by panpipes, a harp or guitar, they conjure up images of a beautiful landscape or a carefree holiday.

Even Gregorian chants are coming back into fashion, as these too have a deep healing effect and let us let go of daily concerns, to relax and be one with the chanting. On your next shopping spree, buy a CD with the singing monks and hear the melodies float from a world of peace beyond space and time. On hearing the garlands of sounds and the power of the calmly flowing male voices, who can help sinking into a splendid state of complete relaxation. In a world of increasing stress, choral singing in its earliest form offers a perfect opportunity for relaxation and moments of happiness.

Baths

Not only in the cold and stressful wintertime but also now and then in other seasons, preferably in the evening, we should treat ourselves to warm and regenerative baths. The moment you step into your bath and lower yourself into the water, you feel its gentle warmth and caress and you scent the added oils. Immersion in the water is a blessing for the senses, so let your body, spirit and soul enjoy it fully. If possible use bath-oils with essential oils added, as pure essential oils are healing and harmonizing. Lavender and balm are calming and relaxing whereas rose and ylang ylang are harmonizing.

Aroma therapy

A special pleasure is afforded by scented lamps impregnated with essential oils. Such an experience fits very nicely into a relaxing evening, when you snugly read a book, meditate or practice yoga. Deeply breathe the aroma of the oils in and focus on the relaxing and harmonizing effect. Some of the oils available are like lavender and balm in being harmonizing, and others are like rose and ylang ylang in being relaxing, so make the best of the qualities of each oil by matching them to your mood.

Oil massages

Massages are among the most effective means of detoxification in helping toxins and slags to be borne away, but they also help to remove psychological burdens and negative memories. Their effects on the whole body are harmonizing and balancing, the body becomes better irrigated with blood, the digestion is stimulated and the muscles are relaxed. Massages are not just a matter of applying the hands in a certain way, to reduce tensions and tallying pains but are also a way to overcome deeper resistance.

If the massage is competent, you head is cleared and your concentration and memory improved, all organs and tissues are rejuvenated and regenerated, the immune system is strengthened and the massage has a liberating, purifying and balancing effect on the mind. All in all, the great benefit is felt by the mind as by the body.

A detoxifying massage is a feast for the senses and has a deep and beneficent effect, countering the effects of stress and dissonance at work. An affectionate massage lets the beneficiary feel the whole force of contact, releasing happiness hormones like serotonin. Owing to the empathetic treatment of the body, tensions and blockages are released and toxins washed away.

The release of blockages and tensions has a positive effect on both physical and psychological ailments. An empathetic massage can arouse a deep feeling of trust towards the masseur, and on the basis of this trust and seclusion, the massage can affect not only the upper layers of tissues but also penetrate deeply into the energy body and soul. False programming of the body can be reached and corrected and the negative effects be removed. With the help of a healing massage, which is much more than a series of grips, a life can be given a fresh direction.

Detoxifying massages mostly involve using a lot of oil, and specifically such harmful substances as are soluble in fat are dissolved then removed from tissues and organs. Some of them are thereby eliminated directly through the skin, especially if warmth is applied. Sweat-cures such as hot, steaming or warm baths following massages widen the pores of the skin and let slag and harmful substances pass through more easily.

Regular movement for activating the lymph

Regular movement not only lets surplus fat melt away, it also improves the metabolism and the circulation of the blood. The improved metabolism is more effective in eliminating slags and toxins, and owing to the improved circulation, more harmful materials can be eliminated through the organs of detoxification and all cells of the body be rejuvenated. Continual movement also helps to lessen stress and to calm the vegetative nervous system.

Lack of movement

The modern way of life is basically static. We travel to work sitting in a car, reach an office by standing in a lift then sit down in the office to have coffee and start work, whereby only a few fingers are active. In earlier days we covered even long distances on foot, and furniture and other accessories were often handmade by the family, not mass produced. These innovations make life easier and health harder, as we move around less and less.

We could compensate for this immobility during the day by moving around more in the evening but seldom do so. Instead of going out to have a stroll through the countryside, we sit down again, to gaze motionlessly at television or at the screen of a computer. We are loath to make even the least physical effort, and only a few of us still do any regular sport, so we just get fatter and feebler.

We are well adapted to natural conditions but not to the conditions which ourselves have created. We evolved to do physical work and to move around on our own two legs. If we finally face up to the fact that we are deteriorating, we react with the same professionalism by driving a few miles to the nearest fitness studio for weight lifting, or we play tennis and end up with tennis-elbow and pains in the knees, since these hobbies are as one-sided as our careers. We then conclude that movement is really no use after all.

So, what can be done to get out of this vicious circle? In fact, we need only keep a few simple rules of suitable movement in mind, then it will benefit all areas of our lives.

Moving the body

Enough physical activity is an important precondition for detoxifying our bodies, strengthening our resilience and creating fresh energy, so it is important to move around daily for awhile, not only briefly. It is also good to do this in the open air in daylight. Open air helps to increase your capacity for oxygen, and daylight to counter any depression. Choose a suitable sport like swimming, walking, hiking or cycling. A further very suitable activity is gardening, as being among plants and flowers is a fine antidote to weariness and exhaustion and alleviates stress and frayed nerves.

Removing toxins

Movement stimulates the circulation of the blood, leading more blood through vessels to organs, whose activity is thereby increased. Blood amply reaches all cells in the body, encouraging rejuvenation and regeneration. Moreover, materials such as toxins, slags and pathogens are thereby moved faster through the lymphatic system and the gut and finally removed.

Movement also stimulates the metabolism of the liver and kidneys, letting them better fulfill their task of detoxification, while dissolved slags and poisons can be washed out of the body faster by the increased flow of blood. Moreover, regular activity also lessens stress, which often besets us everyday at work and gradually depletes our bodies and souls.

Movement out of doors in particular is very useful. Fresh air increases the circulation of the blood, helping the detoxification of the body and especially of the lymph. For improving the health, it is useful to move around out of doors for about 45 minutes 3-5 times per week. Competitive sport should rather be avoided, as it exercises only certain parts of the body, which are thereby not so much regenerated as worn down.

Leisurely sport

The point of leisurely sport is not to move as much as possible as briefly as possible but to move the whole body pleasantly for awhile. Cleaning the windows, mending a fence or raking a garden is more useful than boxing. As far as the task allows, we should perform it with moderate effort for awhile without going so far as to feel signs of strain or exhaustion, since the aim is to let the body regenerate freely. It is also useful to keep to a certain pace and to increase it gradually in the course of time.

Leisurely sport involving the whole body not only increases the metabolism but also the circulation of the blood. The heart is then more efficient and the pulse slower when we are resting. We also become less weighty and ponderous and feel fitter and more mentally balanced, so if we are stressed again, we have more resilience. It is useful to practice at least one leisurely sport, be it hiking, swimming, cycling or dancing, and to change from sport to sport for the sake of variety. The activity should be not only a means to an end but also an end in itself as a pleasant hobby.

On of the best leisurely sports is perfectly simple and can be practiced by nearly everyone. Strolling in the open air calls for no costly equipment, no fitness studio, no elaborate gadgets and no special terrain. Strolling is especially good for training the muscle-vein pump and the lymphatic system. There is no need to rise to the level of jogging but only to cover a fair distance in the open air, and the only equipment needed consists of a pair of suitable shoes and informal clothes, then off you go!

Strolling is good for our bodies in various ways. Moving in the fresh air improves the circulation and detoxification of the body, and variations of temperature and humidity from day to day keep the immune system alert. Hence, you should go out strolling not only on fine days but also on foul ones. As the saying goes, there is no such thing as bad weather, only bad clothing.

If your route is slightly hilly, so much the better, for if your heart beats more noticeably, it is working especially well and will remain more supple and healthy. But a landscape is not only hilly or flat but also a habitat, so viewing various landscapes in the course of the seasons quietens the mind, while the soul rejoices at the sight of nature's variety. On your next stroll, pay more attention to the light and leaves, the scents and sounds and let them work upon you. Watch boughs sway in the breeze, the sun break through a thicket of clouds, and daffodils raise their trumpets to welcome spring. Nature is never the same from day to day.

Dancing

If friends are averse to any kind of activity, dancing is a good way to show them that moving can also be fun and keep the body in form. Dancing is not only a kind of sport but also a means of expression and may be as old as humanity itself. It is also very social, as people literally come into contact with each other, no matter how young or old they happen to be. It is never too late to move to the magic of music and to have fun with a flock of friends.

The whole body is involved in dancing, which is the ideal leisurely sport with a positive effect on the heart and circulatory system, and it also expresses joy. Moving music, a gentle ambiance, elegant clothes and a mischievous glance are a salve for the soul.

Dancing is effective in two respects in detoxifying the body. On the one hand the movement activates the organs of detoxification and on the other hand the feelings experienced in dancing, such as the joy in living, have a positive effect on body and soul, since a relaxed and easygoing person does not accumulate pollutants as much as a tense one. Try the fiery flamingo or classic ballroom dances like the waltz or foxtrot or try racier dances like the salsa and rhumba, to find out which is best for you, then make it your favorite dance and master its steps.

Swimming

This is a very healthy leisurely sport, as we slide and float weightlessly through the water and pleasantly relax. Swimming also detoxifies the body well and stimulates all organs of detoxification, especially the lymphatic system. Aqua-gymnastics and aqua-cycling are likewise good for the lymphatic system, as the pressure of water encourages the flow of lymph. Treading water as advised by Kneipp stimulates lymphatic activity and the removal of stagnant lymph, but you should ensure that the water is not too hot, so it is best to avoid special hot water days or spas with warm water.

Luckily in nearly every town, you can inexpensively practice in indoor swimming pools, but what is more wonderful than to wade into the sea on holiday, to feel its limitless freedom and to view the dome of the sky and the sunshine twinkling on waves?

Cycling

This is a healthy sport for hours at a time and is not only fun but practical for everyone. Cycling is not as demanding as running and strains the heart less, so everyone can go further, even without preparation. Another advantage over running is that joints are flexed even more without having to bear as much weight. It is also a more delightful experience, as you can generally move faster and further and pass through a whole series of scenes. The organs of detoxification are strengthened and supplied with fresh energy, the cardiovascular system is improved, muscles are trained, you lose weight and you are able to do all this while chatting in the company of friends.

On horseback

No other sport brings you closer to nature and lends you a higher vantage point. Swaying and merry on horseback, you have the sportive benefits of riding while viewing the landscape around you, and you may find it easier to ride along sandy paths than to cycle along them. So-called therapeutic riding is also an important way to treat the mentally ill or people with behavioral problems. Riding reawakens all senses, and being so near a fellow creature help a person to be less mentally reserved.

Being walked by a dog

Anyone who is fond of dogs and has enough money and time to look after one should think of buying one. Whatever the weather, a dog will want to go out for a walk and pull you along with him, so you will no longer be able to resort to lazy excuses and instead will be regularly exercised. You will soon forget about life as a lounge lizard and get used to the sun and wind, to rain and snow. Besides, dogs are mostly sociable and keen to get to know other dogs, to you will get to know other humans too. Dogs are also good at relieving you of stress, at calming you down and boosting your sense of security. Stroking a dog may make not only the dog but also you happy, releasing happiness hormones.

Cross-country skiing

What is lovelier than breathing in fresh snowy air and gliding past firs and spruces and quiet woods? Especially in winter, cross-country skiing offers a fine opportunity to lubricate rusty joints and to go out into the hills and woods instead of curling up in front of a fire. Cross-country skiing not only flexes our joints and muscles but also boosts our immune system, to cope with the coming chill. It is the perfect endurance training and is gentle on the joints with little risk of injury. It also positively affects the blood pressure, heart rate and functioning of the lungs.

Epilogue

Never before have we faced as many pollutants as today, whether we willingly absorb them in such forms as alcohol or nicotine or unwillingly in the form of environmental toxins. Besides being exposed to more pollution, our bodies are able to cope with less on account of too little exercise and relaxation and too much unhealthy food.

In principle, our bodies our able to purify and detoxify themselves with the help of several organs with sophisticated mechanisms, but due to the ever-increasing amount of pollution to be disposed of, even the most competent organs are no longer able to cope.

In this situation, it is important to help the organs of detoxification by using measures suitable for increasing their activity, and suitable measures have been outlined above. If the guidance is followed, you may not only be free from illness and pain but also be able to live a more varied, balanced and livelier life.

I hope that this book has been able to give you some valuable tips and suggestions well suited to your needs. Not all these therapies are suited to all readers, but your intuition may lead you to choose well.

I wish you all the best on your personal path to a healthy, happy and eventful life.

Your pharmacist, Angela Fetzner

About the author

Dr. Angela Fetzner was born and grew up in Bad Kissingen in Germany. Since 1996 she has been working as a pharmacist in public and hospital pharmacies, mainly in Germany and Switzerland, and has also held seminars throughout Europe.

She qualified as a pharmacist at the Julius Maximilian University in Würzburg, went on to work for two years in a public pharmacy in the north of Germany and finally undertook postgraduate studies in the history of pharmacy at Philipps University in Marburg, gaining a doctorate (Dr. rer. Nat.).

As a trained pharmacist with useful specialized knowledge, she delights in making complex medical issues widely intelligible and since 2012 has published more than 50 guidebooks and textbooks, many of which are about healthcare and have inspired hundreds of thousands of readers.

In her spare time, she loves to withdraw into nature and to go for long walks with her donkeys, Achiel and Harrie, whom she saved from the slaughterhouse.

A heartfelt thank you

is due at this point to all my esteemed readers. If my guide has been satisfying and useful to you, I would appreciate a short review. Praise, blame or suggestions can be left on my Facebook page:

https://www.facebook.com/AngelaFetzner

or on my homepage as an author:

https://www.angela-fetzner.de

Books from Dr. Angela Fetzner

are likewise all to be found on my homepage as an author:

https://www.angela-fetzner.de

I would also like to offer my readers a special service. My online readings are regularly announced on my homepage, where book reviews and blog articles appear too. On it, you may sign up for my newsletter for regular information about new books, promotions and raffles as well as health tips.

My e-books are in all the leading online stores, and my printed books are in the mail order and standard book trade. I myself am on the social networks: Facebook, Twitter, Instagram and

Youtube: https://angela-fetzner.de//

Your Review and Word-of-Mouth Recommendations Will Make a Difference

Reviews and word-of-mouth recommendations are crucial for any author to succeed. If you enjoyed this book, please leave a review, even if it is only a line or two, and tell your friends about it. It will help the author bring you new books and allow others to also enjoy the book.

Your support is greatly appreciated!

Are You Looking For Other Great Reads?

BABEL
CUBE
BOOKS

Your Books, Your Language

Babelcube Books helps readers find great reads. It plays matchmaker, bringing you and your next book together. Our collection is powered by books produced at Babelcube, a marketplace that brings independent book authors and translators together and distributes their books in multiple languages globally. The books you will find have been translated so that you can discover terrific reads in your language.
We are proud to bring you the world's books.
If you want to learn more about our books, browse our catalog and join our newsletter to learn about our latest releases, visit us at our website:

www.babelcubebooks.com

Made in United States
North Haven, CT
10 November 2026

22095620R10108